ACTIVE YOUTH

Ideas for Implementing CDC Physical Activity Promotion Guidelines

Human Kinetics

Patricia Sammann
Writer

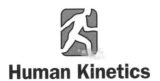

Human Kinetics

Library of Congress Cataloging-in-Publication Data

Active youth : ideas for implementing CDC physical activity promotion
   guidelines / Human Kinetics.
       p.   cm.
   Includes bibliographical references.
   ISBN 0-88011-669-2
   1. Physical education for children--United States--Case studies.
   I. Human Kinetics (Organization)
   GV443.A27   1998
   613.7--dc21

ISBN: 0-88011-669-2   97-17532

Part I, except for the "Recommendations" section, is from the CDC brochure "Guidelines for School and Community Programs to Promote Lifelong Physical Activity Among Young People" by the U.S. Department of Health and Human Services, Centers for Disease Control and Prevention, National Center for Chronic Disease Prevention and Health Promotion, March 1997.

This publication was coordinated through the Association of Teachers of Preventive Medicine (ATPM), and supported by funds from the Centers for Disease Control and Prevention (CDC) under the ATPM/CDC Cooperative Agreement #U50/CCU300860.

CDC Reviewers: Charlene Burgeson, MA; Margaret Davis, MD, MPH; Shannon Paige, MEd; Marlene Tappe (Purdue University), PhD; Howell Wechsler, EdD, MPH; **Acquisitions Editor:** Scott Wikgren; **Developmental Editor:** Holly Gilly; **Managing Editor:** Alesha G. Thompson; **Assistant Editor:** Henry Woolsey; **Editorial Assistants:** Laura Majersky, Amy Carnes, and Erin Sprague; **Copyeditor:** Jim Burns; **Proofreader:** Erin Cler; **Graphic Designer:** Judy Henderson; **Graphic Artist:** Angela K. Snyder and Robert Reuther; **Photo Editor:** Boyd LaFoon; **Cover Designer:** Jack Davis; **Photographer (cover):** © Cheyenne Rouse; **Illustrator:** M.R. Greenberg; **Printer:** United Graphics

Printed in the United States of America

10 9 8 7 6 5 4 3 2 1

Human Kinetics
Web site: http://www.humankinetics.com/

United States: Human Kinetics
P.O. Box 5076
Champaign, IL 61825-5076
1-800-747-4457
e-mail: humank@hkusa.com

Canada: Human Kinetics, Box 24040
Windsor, ON N8Y 4Y9
1-800-465-7301 (in Canada only)
e-mail: humank@hkcanada.com

Europe: Human Kinetics, P.O. Box IW14
Leeds LS16 6TR, United Kingdom
(44) 1132 781708
e-mail: humank@hkeurope.com

Australia: Human Kinetics
57A Price Avenue
Lower Mitcham, South Australia 5062
(088) 277 1555
e-mail: humank@hkaustralia.com

New Zealand: Human Kinetics
P.O. Box 105-231, Auckland 1
(09) 523 3462
e-mail: humank@hknewz.com

Contents

Introduction

Inactivity and poor diet cause more deaths each year in the United States than alcohol, microbial agents, sexual behavior, illicit use of drugs, and firearms *combined!* (McGinnis and Foege, 1993.) Only the use of tobacco is responsible for more preventable deaths (see graph 1). This enormous toll in terms of human life and medical costs illustrates the importance of increasing physical activity levels among both young people and adults.

According to *Physical Activity and Health: A Report of the Surgeon General* (U.S. Department of Health and Human Services 1996), regular physical activity improves health in the following ways:

- Reduces the risk of dying prematurely and dying from heart disease
- Reduces the risk of developing diabetes, high blood pressure, and colon cancer

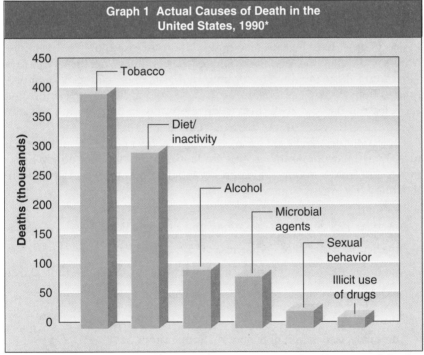

Graph 1 Actual Causes of Death in the United States, 1990*

Note. Data from McGinnis, J.M. and W.H. Foege. 1993. Actual causes of death in the United States. *JAMA*, 18: 2207-12.

* Numbers approximated from various studies that used different approaches to derive estimates.

- Helps reduce blood pressure in people who already have high blood pressure
- Reduces feelings of depression and anxiety and promotes psychological well-being
- Helps control weight
- Helps build and maintain healthy bones, muscles, and joints

DEVELOPING THE GUIDELINES

The Centers for Disease Control and Prevention (CDC), in response to the scientific research regarding the benefits of regular, moderate physical activity, has developed guidelines for increasing physical activity levels among young people. CDC's *Guidelines for School and Community Programs to Promote Lifelong Physical Activity Among Young People,* outline the school and community program strategies that are most likely to be effective in keeping children and adolescents active and preparing them for lifelong participation in physical activity.

These guidelines will be useful to professionals at the national, state, and local levels who design and deliver physical activity programs for young people. They include recommendations relevant to school administrators and policy-makers, classroom teachers, parents, health service providers, and those involved in community-based sport and recreation programs. Policymakers in government and national health and education agencies can use the guidelines to develop new initiatives, and those in higher education can utilize them in training and research.

The guidelines are based on an extensive review of the scientific literature. They incorporate the recommendations from national policy documents and from meetings of experts in the field and representatives from the following organizations:

American Academy of Kinesiology and Physical Education

American Academy of Pediatrics

American Alliance for Health, Physical Education, Recreation and Dance

American Association for Active Lifestyles and Fitness

American Association for Leisure and Recreation

American Association of School Administrators

American College of Sports Medicine

American Federation of Teachers

American Medical Association

American Public Health Association

American School Health Association

Association for the Advancement of Health Education

Council for Exceptional Children

Council of Chief State School Officers

Indian Health Service (Department of Health and Human Services)

National Association for Girls and Women in Sport

National Association for Sport and Physical Education

National Association of Elementary School Principals

National Association of Governor's Councils on Physical Fitness and Sports

National Association of Physical Education in Higher Education

National Association of Secondary School Principals

National Association of State Boards of Education

National Congress of Parents and Teachers

National Dance Association

National Education Association

National Handicapped Sport and Recreation Association

National Heart, Lung and Blood Institute (Department of Health and Human Services)

National Institute for Child Health and Human Development (Department of Health and Human Services)

National Institute of Mental Health (Department of Health and Human Services)

National Recreation and Parks Association

National School Boards Association

National School Health Coalition

President's Council on Physical Fitness and Sports

Society of State Directors of Health, Physical Education, and Recreation

U.S. Department of Education

U.S. Office of Disease Prevention and Health Promotion (Department of Health and Human Services)

Young Men's Christian Associations of the United States of America

Young Women's Christian Association

The following were the technical advisors for *Guidelines for School and Community Programs to Promote Lifelong Physical Activity Among Young People*:

Tom Baranowski, PhD
University of Texas-Houston

Oded Bar-Or, MD
McMaster University

Steven N. Blair, PED
Cooper Institute for Aerobics Research

Charles Corbin, PhD
Arizona State University

Marsha Dowda, MSPH
University of South Carolina

Patty Freedson, PhD
University of Massachusetts

Russell Pate, PhD
University of South Carolina

Sharon Plowman, PhD
Northern Illinois University

James Sallis, PhD
San Diego State University

Ruth Saunders, PhD
University of South Carolina

Vernon Seefeldt, PhD
Michigan State University

Daryl Siedentop, PED
Ohio State University

Bruce Simons-Morton, EdD, MPH
National Institute for Child Health and Human Development

Christine Spain, MA
President's Council on Physical Fitness and Sports

Marlene Tappe, PhD
Centers for Disease Control and Prevention

Dianne Ward, EdD
University of South Carolina

To obtain a complete copy of *Guidelines for School and Community Programs to Promote Lifelong Physical Activity Among Young People,* which includes supporting information and full references, write or call the following:

Centers for Disease Control and Prevention
Division of Adolescent and School Health
Attn: Resource Room
4770 Buford Highway NE
Mailstop K-32
Atlanta, GA 30341-3724
888-CDC-4NRG

To download the guidelines from the Internet, go to **http://www.cdc.gov/nccdphp/dash**. Click on "Strategies" and then select "School Health Programs."

USING THIS BOOK

The book is divided into two parts, the first highlighting the guidelines themselves. There you will find background information on why the guidelines are needed and a complete listing of the guidelines and supporting recommendations. (References have been removed to save space, but are available in the original report.)

The second part of the book presents 20 stories of successful physical activity programs across the country. We chose them to represent a wide range of settings and target audiences in the hope that each reader will find ideas that can be adapted for use in his or her own school or community. Some stories are of school-based programs and some of community organizations; still others are collaborations among several groups. Each story exemplifies implementation of one or more of the guideline recommendations and includes information on how people managed to accomplish this despite facing obstacles similar to the ones you might face in your community.

Each story is assigned a number, and those numbers are listed after the appropriate guidelines at the beginning of part II to indicate which stories cover which guidelines.

Each story talks about how that program began, who started it, and what it took to bring it to life. The stories focus on the practical aspects of program development, from finding money and space to getting support from the community. Roadblocks, successes, and new ideas for making things work are all included.

In most cases these programs have not been subjected to rigorous evaluation and none meet all the guideline recommendations. However, each captures the spirit of some specific guidelines and show resourcefulness in meeting local needs.

Finally, the book ends with a list of agencies and organizations which can provide more specific assistance.

We hope that the guidelines and these real-life examples of their use will inspire you to develop and promote physical activity services for young people in your community. We invite you to draw on the ideas and experience of people around the country who, sometimes with limited money or space, have successfully tackled the problem of creating programs that capture the interest of young people. The future health and fitness of America is at stake, and we all can play a part in seeing that children have the opportunity to develop the skills, confidence, and motivation they need to stay active throughout life.

The Guidelines Explained

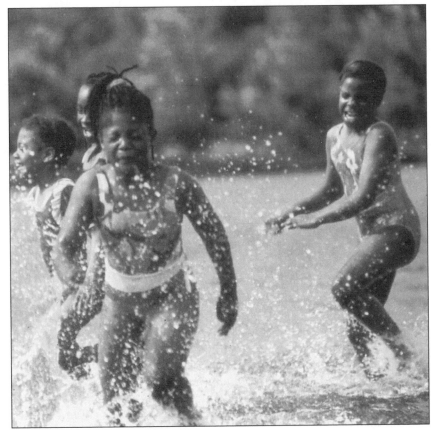

© CLEO Photography

Young people can build healthy bodies and establish healthy lifestyles by including physical activity in their daily lives. However, many young people are not physically active on a regular basis, and physical activity declines dramatically during adolescence. School and community programs can help young people get and stay active, which is why the youth physical activity guidelines were written.

BENEFITS OF PHYSICAL ACTIVITY

Regular physical activity in childhood and adolescence has the following benefits:

- Improves strength and endurance
- Helps build healthy bones and muscles
- Helps control weight
- Reduces anxiety and stress and increases self-esteem
- May improve blood pressure and cholesterol levels

In addition, young people say they like physical activity because it is fun, they do it with friends, and it helps them learn skills, stay in shape, and look better.

Consequences of Physical Inactivity

The long-term consequences of inactivity are serious:

- Inactivity and poor diet cause at least 300,000 deaths a year in the United States. Only tobacco use causes more preventable deaths.
- Adults who are less active are at greater risk of dying of heart disease and developing diabetes, colon cancer, and high blood pressure.

Even during childhood and adolescence, the effects of physical inactivity are evident. As shown in graph 1.1, the percentage of young people who are overweight has more than doubled in the past 30 years.

Physical Activity Among Young People

- Almost half of young people aged 12 to 21 and more than a third of high school students (see graph 1.2) do not participate in vigorous physical activity on a regular basis.
- Seventy-two percent of ninth-graders participate in vigorous physical activity on a regular basis, compared with only 55 percent of twelfth-graders.
- Daily participation in physical education classes by high school students has dropped from 42 percent in 1991 to 25 percent in 1995 (see graph 1.3).

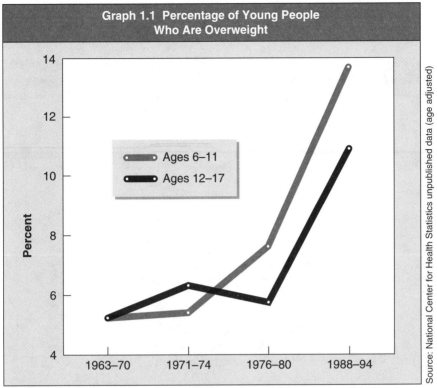

Graph 1.1 Percentage of Young People Who Are Overweight

Legend: Ages 6–11, Ages 12–17

Source: National Center for Health Statistics unpublished data (age adjusted)

Note: Overweight defined by the age- and sex-specific 95th percentile of body mass index from National Health Examination Surveys II and III (1963–70 data).

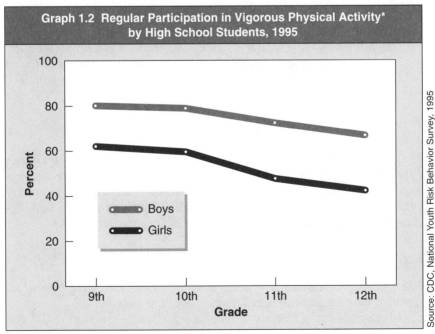

Graph 1.2 Regular Participation in Vigorous Physical Activity* by High School Students, 1995

Legend: Boys, Girls

Source: CDC, National Youth Risk Behavior Survey, 1995

*On 3 or more of the 7 days preceding the survey, at least 20 minutes participation in activities that made the students breathe hard and sweat.

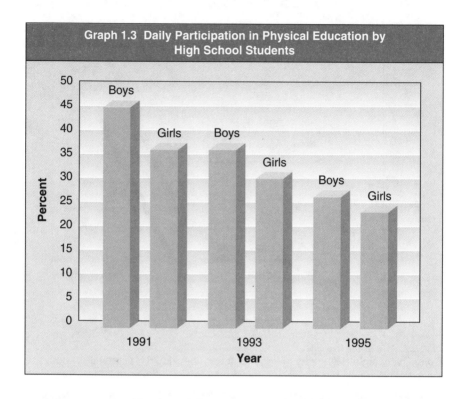

Graph 1.3 Daily Participation in Physical Education by High School Students

- The time students spend being active in physical education classes is decreasing. Among high school students enrolled in a physical education class, the percentage who were active for at least 20 minutes during an average class dropped from 81 percent in 1991 to 70 percent in 1995.

THE CDC'S GUIDELINES

The CDC's *Guidelines for School and Community Programs to Promote Lifelong Physical Activity Among Young People* were developed in collaboration with experts from other federal agencies, state agencies, universities, voluntary organizations, and professional organizations. They are based on an extensive review of research and practice.

Key Principles

The guidelines state that physical activity programs for young people are most likely to be effective when they do the following:

- Emphasize enjoyable participation in physical activities that are easily done throughout life
- Offer a diverse range of noncompetitive and competitive activities appropriate for different ages and abilities
- Give young people the skills and confidence they need to be physically active
- Promote physical activity through all components of a coordinated school health program and develop links between school and community programs

How Much Physical Activity Do Young People Need?

Everyone can benefit from a moderate amount of physical activity on most, if not all, days of the week. Young people should select activities they enjoy that fit into their daily lives. Examples of moderate activity include the following:

- Walking two miles in 30 minutes or running one and a half miles in 15 minutes

- Bicycling five miles in 30 minutes or four miles in 15 minutes

- Dancing fast for 30 minutes or jumping rope for 15 minutes

- Playing basketball for 15 to 20 minutes or volleyball for 45 minutes

(For more examples of moderate physical activities, see figure 1.1.)
  Increasing the frequency, time, or intensity of physical activity can bring even more health benefits—up to a point. Too much physical activity can lead to injuries and other health problems.

Recommendations

The guidelines include 10 main recommendations for ensuring quality physical activity programs, along with supporting recommendations for each.

1. **Policy:** Establish policies that promote enjoyable, lifelong physical activity among young people.
2. **Environment:** Provide physical and social environments that encourage and enable safe and enjoyable physical activity.

Figure 1.1 Examples of Moderate Amounts of Activity

Washing and waxing a car for 45–60 minutes

Washing windows or floors for 45–60 minutes

Playing volleyball for 45 minutes

Playing touch football for 30–45 minutes

Gardening for 30–45 minutes

Wheeling self in wheelchair for 30–40 minutes

Walking 1¾ miles in 35 minutes (20 min/mile)

Basketball (shooting baskets) for 30 minutes

Bicycling 5 miles in 30 minutes

Dancing fast (social) for 30 minutes

Pushing a stroller 1½ miles in 30 minutes

Raking leaves for 30 minutes

Walking 2 miles in 30 minutes (15 min/mile)

Water aerobics for 30 minutes

Swimming laps for 20 minutes

Wheelchair basketball for 20 minutes

Basketball (playing a game) for 15–20 minutes

Bicycling 4 miles in 15 minutes

Jumping rope for 15 minutes

Running 1½ miles in 15 minutes (10 min/mile)

Shoveling snow for 15 minutes

Stairwalking for 15 minutes

Less vigorous, more time ↑ ↓ *More vigorous, less time*

Note: A moderate amount of physical activity is roughly equivalent to physical activity that uses approximately 150 calories (kcal) of energy per day, or 1,000 calories per week. Some activities can be performed at various intensities; the suggested durations correspond to expected intensity of effort.

3. **Physical education:** Implement physical education curricula and instruction that emphasize enjoyable participation in physical activity and that help students develop the knowledge, attitudes, motor skills, behavioral skills, and confidence needed to adopt and maintain physically active lifestyles.

4. **Health education:** Implement health education curricula and instruction that help students develop the knowledge, attitudes, behavioral skills, and confidence needed to adopt and maintain physically active lifestyles.

5. **Extracurricular activities:** Provide extracurricular physical activity programs that meet the needs and interests of all students.

6. **Parental involvement:** Include parents and guardians in physical activity instruction and in extracurricular and community physical

activity programs, and encourage them to support their children's participation in enjoyable physical activities.

7. **Personnel training:** Provide training for education, coaching, recreation, health-care, and other school and community personnel that imparts the knowledge and skills needed to effectively promote enjoyable, lifelong physical activity among young people.

8. **Health services:** Assess physical activity patterns among young people, counsel them about physical activity, refer them to appropriate programs, and advocate for physical activity instruction and programs for them.

9. **Community programs:** Provide a range of developmentally appropriate community sports and recreation programs that are attractive to all young people.

10. **Evaluation:** Regularly evaluate school and community physical activity instruction, programs, and facilities.

1 POLICY

Establish policies that promote enjoyable, lifelong physical activity among young people.

Policies provide formal and informal rules that guide schools and communities in planning, implementing, and evaluating physical activity programs for young people. School and community policies related to physical activity should comply with state and local laws and with recommendations and standards provided by national, state, and local agencies and organizations. These policies should be included in a written document that incorporates input from administrators, teachers, coaches, athletic trainers, parents, students, health-care providers, public health professionals, and other school and community personnel, and should address the following requirements.

Require comprehensive, daily physical education for students in kindergarten through grade 12.

Physical education instruction can increase students' knowledge, physical activity, and physical fitness. Daily physical education from kindergarten through 12th grade is recommended by the American Heart Association and the National Association for Sport and Physical Education, and is also a national health objective for the year 2000. The minimum amount of physical education required for students is usually set by state law. Although most states (94 percent) and school districts (95 percent) require some physical education, only one state requires it daily from kindergarten through 12th grade. Less than two-thirds (60 percent) of high school students are

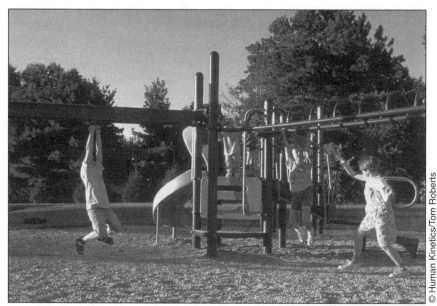

Space for physical activity should be available to young people before, during, and after the school day and on weekends and during the summer.

enrolled in physical education classes, and only 25 percent take physical education daily. Enrollment in both physical education (9th grade, 81 percent; 12th grade, 42 percent) and daily physical education (9th grade, 41 percent; 12th grade, 13 percent) declines in higher grades, and enrollment in daily physical education and active time in physical education classes decreased among high school students from 1991 to 1995. Further, 30 percent of schools exempt students from physical education if they participate in band, chorus, cheerleading, or interscholastic sports. Substitution of these programs for physical education reduces students' opportunities to develop knowledge, attitudes, motor skills, behavioral skills, and confidence related to physical activity.

Require comprehensive health education for students in kindergarten through grade 12.

Comprehensive health education, which includes instruction on physical activity topics, can complement the instruction students receive in comprehensive physical education. Health education may improve students' health knowledge, attitudes, and behaviors. Many educational organizations recommend that students receive planned and sequential health education from kindergarten through 12th grade, and such education is a national health objective for the year 2000. Although 90 percent of states and 91 percent of school districts require that schools offer health education, fewer school districts require that a separate course be devoted to health topics (elementary school, 19 percent; middle school, 44 percent; senior high school, 66 percent). Administrators of public schools and parents of adolescents in public schools believe that these students should be taught more health information and skills.

Require that adequate resources, including budget and facilities, be committed for physical activity instruction and programs.

The National Association for Sport and Physical Education and the Joint Committee for National Health Education Standards note that adequate budget and facilities are necessary for physical education, health education, extracurricular physical activities, and community sports and recreation programs to be successful. However, these programs rarely have sufficient resources. Schools and communities should be vigilant in making sure that physical education, health education, and physical activity programs have sufficient financial and facility resources to ensure safe participation by young people. Schools should have policies that ensure that teacher-to-student ratios in physical education are comparable to those in other subjects and that physical education spaces and facilities are not usurped for other events. Schools should have policies requiring that physical education classes be scheduled so that students in each class are of similar physical maturity and grade level.

Require the hiring of physical education specialists to teach physical education in kindergarten through grade 12, elementary school teachers trained to teach health education, health education specialists to teach health education in middle and senior high schools, and qualified people to direct school and community physical activity programs and to coach young people in sports and recreation programs.

Planning, implementing, and evaluating physical activity instruction and programs require specially trained personnel. Physical education specialists teach longer lessons, spend more time on developing skills, impart more knowledge, and provide more moderate and vigorous physical activity than do classroom teachers. Schools should have policies requiring that physical education specialists teach physical education in kindergarten through grade 12, elementary school teachers trained to teach health education do so in elementary schools, health education specialists teach health education in middle and senior high schools, and qualified people direct school and community physical activity programs and coach young people in sports and recreation programs.

Some states have established minimum standards for teachers. Eighty-four percent of states require physical education certification for secondary school physical education teachers, and 16 percent require such certification for elementary school physical education teachers. Only 69 percent of states require health education certification for secondary school health education teachers. These data indicate the need for a greater commitment to hiring professionally trained physical education and health education specialists for our nation's schools.

Some states have established minimum standards for athletic coaches. Both schools and communities should have policies that require employing people who have the coaching competency appropriate to participants' developmental and skill levels. Coaches who work with beginning athletes should meet at least the Level I, if not Level II, coaching competencies identified by the National Association for Sport and Physical Education. Entry-level interscholastic coaches and master coaches should achieve at least Level III and Level IV coaching competencies, respectively.

Require that physical activity instruction and programs meet the needs and interests of all students.

All students, irrespective of their sex, race/ethnicity, health status, or physical and cognitive ability or disability should have access to physical education, health education, extracurricular physical activity programs, and community sports and recreation programs that meet their needs and interests. In addition, physical activity programs that overemphasize a limited set of team sports and underemphasize noncompetitive, lifetime fitness and recreational activities (e.g., walking or bicycling) could exclude or be unattractive to potential participants.

Adolescents' interests and participation in physical activity differ by sex. For example, compared with boys, girls engage in less physical activity, are less likely to participate in team sports, and are more likely to participate in aerobics or dance. Girls and boys also perceive different benefits of physical activity; for example, boys more often cite competition and girls more often cite weight management as a reason for engaging in physical activity. Because boys are more likely than girls to have higher perceptions of self-efficacy and physical competence, physical activity programs serving girls should provide instruction and experiences that increase girls' confidence in participating in physical activity, opportunities for them to participate in physical activities, and social environments that support their involvement in a range of physical activities. Adolescents' participation in physical activity also differs by race and ethnicity.

Children and adolescents who are obese or who have physical or cognitive disabilities, chronic health conditions (e.g., diabetes, heart disease, or asthma), or low levels of fitness need instruction and programs in which they can develop motor skills, improve fitness, and experience enjoyment and success. Young people who have these disabilities or health concerns are often overtly or unintentionally discouraged from engaging in regular physical activity even though they may be in particular need of it. For example, 59 percent of high schools allow students who have physical disabilities to be exempt from physical education courses. Schools should be required to provide modified physical education and health education for these students. By modifying physical education, health education, extracurricular physical activities, and community sports and recreation programs, schools and communities can help these young people acquire the physical, mental, and social benefits of physical activity.

Physical education, health education, extracurricular physical activity programs, and community sports and recreation programs can also provide opportunities for multicultural experiences (e.g., American Indian and African dance). These experiences can meet children's and adolescents' interests and foster their awareness and appreciation of physical activities enjoyed by different cultural groups.

2 ENVIRONMENT

Provide physical and social environments that encourage and enable safe and enjoyable physical activity.

The physical and social environments of children and adolescents should encourage and enable their participation in safe and enjoyable physical activities. These environments are described by the following guidelines.

Provide access to safe spaces and facilities for physical activity in the school and the community.

School spaces and facilities should be available to young people before, during, and after the school day, on weekends, and during summer and other vacations. These spaces and facilities should also be readily available to community agencies and organizations offering physical activity programs.

National health objective 1.11 calls for increased availability of facilities for physical activity (e.g., hiking, bicycling, and fitness trails; public swimming pools; and parks and open spaces for recreation). Community coalitions should coordinate the availability of these open spaces and facilities. Some communities may need to build new facilities, whereas others may need only to coordinate existing community spaces and facilities. The needs of all children and adolescents, particularly those who have disabilities, should be incorporated into the building of new facilities and the coordination of existing ones.

Schools and communities should ensure that spaces and facilities meet or exceed recommended safety standards for design, installation, and maintenance. For example, playgrounds should have cool water and adequate shade for play and rest. Young people also need places that are free from violence and free from exposure to environmental hazards such as fumes from incinerators or motor vehicles. Spaces and facilities for physical activity should be regularly inspected, and hazardous conditions should be immediately corrected.

Establish and enforce measures to prevent physical activity–related injuries and illnesses.

Minimizing physical activity–related injuries and illnesses among young people is the joint responsibility of teachers, administrators, coaches, athletic trainers, other school and community personnel, parents, and young people. Preventing injuries and illness includes having appropriate adult supervision, complying with safety rules and the use of protective clothing and equipment, and avoiding the effects of extreme weather conditions. Explicit safety rules should be taught to, and followed by, young people in physical education, health education, extracurricular physical activity programs, and community sports and recreation programs. Adult supervisors should consistently reinforce safety rules.

Adult supervisors should be aware of the potential for physical activity–related injuries and illnesses among young people so that the risks for and consequences of these injuries and illnesses can be minimized. These adults should receive medical information relevant to each student's participation in physical activity (e.g., whether the child has asthma), be able to provide first aid and cardiopulmonary resuscitation, and practice precautions to prevent the spread of bloodborne pathogens such as the human immunodeficiency virus. Written policies on providing first aid and reporting injuries and illnesses to parents and to appropriate school and community authorities should be established and followed. Adult supervisors can take the following steps to avoid injuries and illnesses during structured physical activity for young people: require physical assessment before participation, provide developmentally appropriate activities, ensure proper conditioning, provide instruction on the biomechanics of specific motor skills, appropriately match participants according to size and ability, adapt rules to the skill level of young people and the protective equipment available, avoid excesses in training, modify rules to eliminate unsafe practices, and ensure that injuries are healed before further participation.

Children and adolescents should be provided with, and required to use, protective clothing and equipment appropriate to the type of physical activity and the environment. Protective clothing and equipment includes footwear appropriate for the specific activity; helmets for bicycling; helmets, face masks, mouthguards, and protective pads for football and ice hockey; and reflective clothing for walking and running. Protective gear and athletic equipment should be frequently inspected, and they should be replaced if worn, damaged, or outdated.

Exposure to the sun can be minimized by use of protective hats, clothing, and sunscreen; avoidance of midday sun exposure; and use of shaded spaces or indoor facilities. Heat-related illnesses can be prevented by ensuring that children and adolescents frequently drink cool water, have adequate rest and shade, play during cool times of the day, and are supervised by people trained to recognize the early signs of heat exhaustion and heatstroke. Cold-related injuries can be avoided by making sure that young people wear multilayered clothing for outside play and exercise, increasing the intensity of outdoor activities, using indoor facilities during extremely cold weather, ensuring proper water temperature for aquatic activities, and providing supervision by people trained to recognize the early signs of frostbite and hypothermia. Measures such as reducing the intensity of physical activity or holding physical education classes or programs indoors should be taken to avoid health problems associated with poor air quality .

Teachers, parents, coaches, athletic trainers, and health-care providers should promote a range of healthy behaviors. These adults should encourage young people to abstain from tobacco, alcohol, and other drugs; maintain a healthy diet; and practice healthy weight-management techniques. Adult supervisors should be aware of the signs and symptoms of eating disorders and take steps to prevent eating disorders among young people.

Provide time within the school day for unstructured physical activity.

During the school day, opportunities for physical activity exist within physical education classes, during recess, and immediately before and after school. For example, students in grades one through four have an average recess period of 30 minutes. School personnel should encourage students to be physically active during these times. The use of time during the school day for unstructured physical activity should complement rather than substitute for the physical activity and instruction children receive in physical education classes.

Discourage the use or withholding of physical activity as punishment.

Teachers, coaches, and other school and community personnel should not force participation in, or withhold opportunities for, physical activity as punishment. Using physical activity as a punishment risks creating negative associations with physical activity in the minds of young people. Withholding physical activity deprives students of health benefits important to their well-being.

Provide health promotion programs for school faculty and staff.

Enabling school personnel to participate in physical activity and other healthy behaviors should help them serve as role models for students. School-based health promotion programs have been effective in improving teachers' participation in vigorous exercise, which in turn has improved their physical fitness, body composition, blood pressure, general well-being, and ability to handle job stress. In addition, participants in school-based health promotion programs may be less likely than nonparticipants to be absent from work.

3 PHYSICAL EDUCATION

Implement physical education curricula and instruction that emphasize enjoyable participation in physical activity and that help students develop the knowledge, attitudes, motor skills, behavioral skills, and confidence needed to adopt and maintain physically active lifestyles.

Physical education curricula and instruction are vital parts of a comprehensive school health program. One of the main goals of these curricula should be to help students develop an active lifestyle that will persist into and throughout adulthood.

Provide planned and sequential physical education curricula from kindergarten through grade 12 that promote enjoyable, lifelong physical activity.

School physical education curricula are often mandated by state laws or regulations. Many states (76 percent) and school districts (89 percent) have written goals, objectives, or outcomes for physical education, and only 26 percent of states require a senior high school physical education course promoting physical activities that can be enjoyed throughout life. Planned and sequential physical education curricula should emphasize knowledge about the benefits of physical activity and the recommended amounts and types of physical activity needed to promote health. Physical education should help students develop the attitudes, motor skills, behavioral skills, and confidence they need to engage in lifelong physical activity. Physical education should emphasize skills for lifetime physical activities (e.g., dance, strength training, jogging, swimming, bicycling, cross-country skiing, walking, and hiking) rather than those for competitive sports.

If physical fitness testing is used, it should be integrated into the curriculum and emphasize health-related components of physical fitness (e.g., cardiorespiratory endurance, muscular strength and endurance, flexibility, and body composition). The tests should be administered only after students are well oriented to the testing procedures. Testing should be a mechanism for teaching students how to apply behavioral skills (e.g., self-assessment, goal setting, and self-monitoring) to physical fitness development and for providing feedback to students and parents about students'

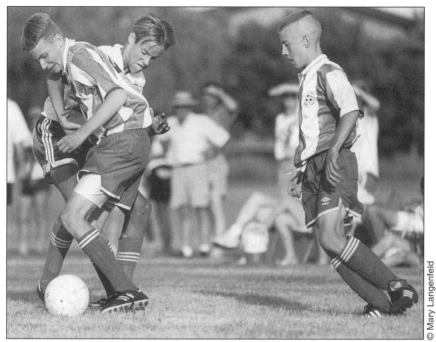

© Mary Langenfeld

Steps, such as ensuring proper conditioning and appropriately matching participants according to size and ability, should be taken to avoid injuries during structured physical activity for young people.

physical fitness. The results of physical fitness testing should not be used to assign report card grades. Also, test results should not be used to assess program effectiveness; the validity of these measurements may be unreliable, and physical fitness and improvements in physical fitness are influenced by factors (e.g., physical maturation, body size, and body composition) beyond the control of teachers and students.

Use physical education curricula consistent with the national standards for physical education.

The national standards for physical education describe what students should know and be able to do as a result of physical education. A student educated about physical activity "has learned skills necessary to perform a variety of physical activities, is physically fit, does participate regularly in physical activity, knows the implications of and the benefits from involvement in physical activities, [and] values physical activity and its contribution to a healthful lifestyle." The national standards emphasize the development of movement competency and proficiency, use of cognitive information to enhance motor skill acquisition and performance, establishment of regular participation in physical activity, achievement of health-enhancing physical fitness, development of responsible personal and social behavior, understanding of and respect for individual differences, and awareness of values and benefits of physical activity participation. These standards provide a framework that should be used to design, implement, and evaluate physical education curricula that promote enjoyable, lifelong physical activity.

Use active learning strategies and emphasize enjoyable participation in physical education class.

Enjoyable physical education experiences are believed to be essential in promoting physical activity among children and adolescents. Physical education experiences that are enjoyable and actively involve students in learning may help foster positive attitudes toward and encourage participation in physical education and physical activity. Active learning strategies that involve the student in learning physical activity concepts, motor skills, and behavioral skills include brainstorming, cooperative groups, simulation, and situation analysis.

Develop students' knowledge of and positive attitudes toward physical activity.

Knowledge of physical activity is viewed as an essential component of physical education curricula. Related concepts include the physical, social, and mental health benefits of physical activity; the components of health-related fitness; principles of exercise; injury prevention; precautions for preventing the spread of bloodborne pathogens; nutrition and weight management; social influences on physical activity; and the development of safe and effective individualized physical activity programs. For both young people and adults, knowledge about *how* to be physically active may be a more important influence on physical activity than knowledge about *why* to be active.

Positive attitudes toward physical activity may affect young people's involvement in it. Positive attitudes include perceptions that physical activity is important and that it is fun. Ways to generate positive attitudes include providing students with enjoyable physical education experiences that meet their needs and interests, emphasizing the many benefits of physical activity, supporting students who are physically active, and using active learning strategies.

Develop students' mastery of and confidence in motor and behavioral skills for participating in physical activity.

Physical education should help students master and gain confidence in motor and behavioral skills used in physical activity. Students should become competent in many motor skills and proficient in a few to use in lifelong physical activities. Elementary school students should develop basic motor skills that allow participation in a variety of physical activities, and older students should become competent in a select number of lifetime physical activities they enjoy and succeed in. Students' mastery of and confidence in motor skills occurs when these skills are broken down into components and the tasks are ordered from easy to hard. In addition, students need opportunities to observe others performing the skills and to receive encouragement, feedback, and repeated opportunities for practice during physical education class.

Behavioral skills (e.g., self-assessment, self-monitoring, decision making, goal setting, and communication) may help students establish and maintain regular involvement in physical activity. Active student involvement and social learning experiences that focus on building confidence may increase the likelihood that children and adolescents will enjoy and succeed in physical education and physical activity.

Provide a substantial percentage of each student's recommended weekly amount of physical activity in physical education classes.

For physical education to make a meaningful and consistent contribution to the recommended amount of young people's physical activity, students at every grade level should take physical education classes that meet daily and should be physically active for a large percentage of class time. National health objective 1.9 calls for students to be physically active for at least 50 percent of physical education class time, but many schools do not meet this objective, and the percentage of time students spend in moderate or vigorous physical activity during physical education classes has decreased over the past few years.

Promote participation in enjoyable physical activity in the school, community, and home.

Physical education teachers should encourage students to be active before, during, and after the school day. Physical education teachers can also refer students to sports and recreation programs available in their community and promote participation in physical activity at home by assigning homework that students can do on their own or with family members.

4   HEALTH EDUCATION

Implement health education curricula and instruction that help students develop the knowledge, attitudes, behavioral skills, and confidence needed to adopt and maintain physically active lifestyles.

Health education can effectively promote students' health-related knowledge, attitudes, and behaviors. The major contribution of health education in promoting physical activity among students should be to help them develop the knowledge, attitudes, and behavioral skills they need to establish and maintain a physically active lifestyle.

Provide planned and sequential health education curricula from kindergarten through grade 12 that promote lifelong participation in physical activity.

Many states (65 percent) and school districts (82 percent) require that physical activity and physical fitness topics be part of a required course in health education. Planned and sequential health education curricula, like physical education curricula, should draw on social cognitive theory and emphasize physical activity as a component of a healthy lifestyle.

Use health education curricula consistent with the national standards for health education.

The national standards for health education developed by the Joint Committee on National Health Education Standards describe what health-literate students should know and be able to do as a result of school health education. Health literacy is "the capacity of individuals to obtain, interpret, and understand basic health information and services and the competence to use such information and services in ways which enhance health." The standards specify that, as a result of health education, students should be able to comprehend basic health concepts; access valid health information and health-promoting products and services; practice health-enhancing behaviors; analyze the influence of culture and other factors on health; use interpersonal communication skills to enhance health; use goal-setting and decision-making skills to enhance health; and advocate for personal, family, and community health. These standards emphasize the development of students' skills and can be used as the basis for health education curricula.

Promote collaboration among physical education, health education, and classroom teachers as well as teachers in related disciplines who plan and implement physical activity instruction.

Physical education and health education teachers in about one-third of middle and senior high schools collaborate on activities or projects. Collaboration allows coordinated physical activity instruction and should enable teachers to provide range and depth of physical activity–related content and skills. For example, health education and physical education teachers can collaborate to reinforce the link between sound dietary practices and regular physical activity for weight management. Collaboration also allows teachers to highlight the influence of behaviors such as using alcohol or other drugs on the capacity to engage in physical activity, or behaviors such as not using tobacco that interact with physical activity to reduce the risk of developing chronic diseases.

Use active learning strategies to emphasize enjoyable participation in physical activity in the school, community, and home.

Health education instruction should include the use of active learning strategies. Such strategies may encourage students' active involvement in learning and help them develop the concepts, attitudes, and behavioral skills they need to engage in physical activity. Additionally, health education teachers should encourage students to adopt healthy behaviors (e.g., physical activity) in the school, community, and home.

Develop students' knowledge of and positive attitudes toward healthy behaviors, particularly physical activity.

Health education curricula should provide information about physical activity concepts. These concepts should include the physical, social, and mental health benefits of physical activity; the components of health-related fitness; principles of exercise; injury prevention and first aid; precautions for preventing the spread of bloodborne pathogens; nutrition, physical activity, and weight management; social influences on physical activity; and the development of safe and effective individualized physical activity programs.

Health instruction should also generate positive attitudes toward healthy behaviors. These positive attitudes include perceptions that it is important and fun to participate in physical activity. Ways to foster positive attitudes include emphasizing the multiple benefits of physical activity, supporting children and adolescents who are physically active, and using active learning strategies.

Develop students' mastery of and confidence in the behavioral skills needed to adopt and maintain a healthy lifestyle that includes regular physical activity.

Children and adolescents should develop behavioral skills that may enable them to adopt healthy behaviors. Certain skills (e.g., self-assessment, self-monitoring, decision making, goal setting, identifying and managing barriers, self-regulation, reinforcement, communication, and advocacy) may help students adopt and maintain a healthy lifestyle that includes regular physical activity. Active learning strategies give students opportunities to practice, master, and develop confidence in these skills.

5 EXTRACURRICULAR ACTIVITIES

Provide extracurricular physical activity programs that meet the needs and interests of all students.

Extracurricular activities are any activities offered by schools outside of formal classes. Interscholastic athletics, intramural sports, and sports and recreation clubs are believed to contribute to the physical and social development of young people, and schools should extend these benefits to the greatest possible number of students. These activities can help meet the goals of comprehensive school health programs by providing students with opportunities to engage in physical activity and to further develop the knowledge, attitudes, motor and behavioral skills, and confidence needed to adopt and maintain physically active lifestyles.

Provide a diversity of developmentally appropriate competitive and noncompetitive physical activity programs for all students.

Interscholastic athletic programs are typically limited to the secondary school level and usually consist of a few highly competitive team sports. Intramural sports programs are not common but, where they are offered, usually emphasize competitive team sports. Such programs usually underserve students who are less skilled, less physically fit, or not attracted to competitive sports. One reason that participation in sports declines steadily during late childhood and adolescence is that undue emphasis is placed on competition.

After the needs and interests of all students are assessed, interscholastic, intramural, and club programs should be modified and expanded to offer a range of competitive and noncompetitive activities. For example, noncompetitive lifetime physical activities include walking, running, swimming, and bicycling.

Link students to community physical activity programs, and use community resources to support extracurricular physical activity programs.

Schools should work with community organizations to enhance the appropriate use of out-of-school time among children and adolescents and to develop effective systems for referring young people from schools to community agencies and organizations that can provide needed services. To help students learn about community resources, schools can sponsor information fairs that represent community groups; physical education and health education teachers can provide information about community resources as part of the curricula; and community-based program personnel can be speakers or demonstration lecturers in school classes.

Frequently schools have the facilities but lack the personnel to deliver extracurricular physical activity programs. Community resources can expand existing school programs by providing intramural and club activities on school grounds. For example, community agencies and organizations can use school facilities for after-school physical fitness programs for children and adolescents, weight-management programs for overweight or obese young people, and sports and recreation programs for young people with disabilities or chronic health conditions.

6 PARENTAL INVOLVEMENT

Include parents and guardians in physical activity instruction and in extracurricular and community physical activity programs, and encourage them to support their children's participation in enjoyable physical activities.

Parental involvement in children's physical activity instruction and programs is key to the development of a psychosocial environment that promotes physical activity among young people. Involvement in these programs provides parents opportunities to be partners in developing their children's physical activity–related knowledge, attitudes, motor and behavioral skills, confidence, and behavior. Thus, teachers, coaches, and other school and community personnel should encourage and enable parental involvement. For example, teachers can assign homework to students that must be done with their parents and can provide flyers designed for parents that contain information and strategies for promoting physical activity within the family. Parents can also join school health advisory councils, booster clubs, and parent-teacher organizations. Parents who have been trained by professionals can also serve as volunteer coaches for or leaders of extracurricular physical activity programs and community sports and recreation programs.

Encourage parents to advocate for quality physical activity instruction and programs for their children.

Parents may be able to influence the quality and quantity of physical activity available to their children by advocating for comprehensive, daily

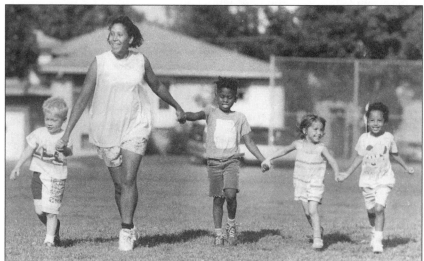

Parents who have been trained by professionals can serve as volunteer coaches or leaders of extracurricular physical activity programs.

physical education in schools and for school and community physical activity programs that promote lifelong physical activity among young people. Parents should also advocate for safe spaces and facilities that provide their children opportunities to engage in a range of physical activities.

Encourage parents to support their children's participation in appropriate, enjoyable physical activities.

Parents should ensure that their children participate in physical education classes, extracurricular physical activity programs, and community sports and recreation programs in which the children will experience enjoyment and success. Parents should learn what their children want from extracurricular and community physical activity programs and then help select appropriate activities. Fun and skill development, rather than winning, are the primary reasons most young people participate in physical activity and sports programs. Parents should help their children gain access to toys and equipment for physical activity and transportation to activity sites.

Encourage parents to be physically active role models and to plan and participate in family activities that include physical activity.

Parental support is a determinant of physical activity among children and adolescents, and parents' attitudes may influence children's involvement. Parents and guardians should try to be role models for physical activity behavior and should plan and participate in family activities such as going to the community swimming pool or using the community trails for bicycling or walking.

Because peers and friends influence children's physical activity behavior, parents can encourage their children to be active with their friends. Children's participation in sedentary activities (e.g., watching television or playing video games) should be monitored and replaced with physical activity, and parents should encourage their children to play outside in supervised playgrounds and parks and other safe places.

7 PERSONNEL TRAINING

Provide training for education, coaching, recreation, health-care, and other school and community personnel that imparts the knowledge and skills needed to effectively promote enjoyable, lifelong physical activity among young people.

The lack of trained personnel is a barrier to implementing safe, organized, and effective physical activity instruction and programs for young people.

National, state, and local education and health agencies; institutions of higher education; and national and state professional organizations should collaborate to provide teachers, coaches, administrators, and other school personnel preservice and in-service training in promoting enjoyable, lifelong physical activity among young people. Instructor training has proven to be efficacious; for example, physical education specialists teach longer and higher quality lessons, and teacher training is important in successful implementation of innovative health education curricula. Institutions of higher education should use national guidelines such as those for athletic coaches, entry-level physical education teachers, entry-level health education teachers, and elementary school classroom teachers to plan, implement, and evaluate professional preparation programs for school personnel. In addition, physicians, school nurses, and others who provide health services to young people need preservice training in promoting physical activity and providing physical activity assessment, counseling, and referral.

Although 72 percent of states and 50 percent of school districts provide in-service training on physical education topics, all states and school districts need to do so. School personnel often want more training than they receive. For example, more than one-third of lead physical education teachers want additional training in developing individualized fitness programs, increasing students' physical activity inside and outside of class, and involving families in physical activity.

Train teachers to deliver physical education that provides a substantial percentage of each student's recommended weekly amount of physical activity.

The proportion of physical education class time spent on moderate or vigorous physical activity is insufficient to meet national health objective 1.9. In-service teacher training that focuses on increasing the amount of class time spent on moderate or vigorous physical activity is effective in increasing students' physical activity during physical education classes. Although 52 percent of states have offered training to physical education teachers on increasing students' physical activity during class, only 15 percent of school districts have provided this training. National, state, and local education and health agencies; institutions of higher education; and national and state professional organizations should augment efforts to provide this training to teachers.

Train teachers to use active learning strategies needed to develop students' knowledge about, attitudes toward, skills in, and confidence in engaging in physical activity.

Physical education and health education teachers should observe experienced teachers using active learning strategies, have hands-on practice in using these strategies, and receive feedback. Such training should increase teachers' use of these strategies.

Train school and community personnel how to create psychosocial environments that enable young people to enjoy physical activity instruction and programs.

Preservice and in-service training should help teachers, coaches, and other school and community personnel plan and implement physical education as well as extracurricular and community physical activity programs that meet a range of students' needs and interests. Training should also encourage these school and community personnel to place less emphasis on competition and more emphasis on students' having fun and developing skills.

Train school and community personnel how to involve parents and the community in physical activity instruction and programs.

Few teachers, coaches, and other school personnel have been trained to involve families and the community in physical activity instruction and programs. Instruction on communication skills for interacting with parents and the community as well as strategies for obtaining adults' support for physical activity instruction and programs is beneficial. Teachers should have the knowledge, skills, and materials for creating fact sheets for parents and assigning physical education and health education homework for students to complete with their families.

Train volunteers who coach sports and recreation programs for young people.

Volunteer coaches who work with beginning athletes in schools and communities should have the level coaching competency delineated by the National Association for Sport and Physical Education. Like professional coaches, volunteer coaches should receive professional training on how to provide experiences for young people that emphasize fun, skill development, confidence-building, self-knowledge and injury prevention, first aid, cardiopulmonary resuscitation, precautions against contamination by bloodborne pathogens, and promotion of other healthy behaviors (e.g., dietary behavior).

8 HEALTH SERVICES

Assess physical activity patterns among young people, counsel them about physical activity, refer them to appropriate programs, and advocate for physical activity instruction and programs for them.

Physicians, school nurses, and other people who provide health services to young people have a key role in promoting healthy behaviors. Health-care providers are important in promoting physical activity, especially among children and adolescents who have physical and cognitive disabilities or chronic health conditions.

Regularly assess the physical activity patterns of young people, reinforce physical activity among active young people, counsel inactive young people about physical activity, and refer young people to appropriate physical activity programs.

As a routine part of care, health-care providers should assess the physical activity of their young patients. Young people and their families should be counseled about the importance of physical activity and be provided information that enables them to initiate and maintain regular, safe, and enjoyable participation in physical activity. Children and adolescents who are already active should be encouraged to continue their physical activity. Health-care providers should work with inactive young people and their families to develop exercise prescriptions and should refer these young people to school and community physical activity programs appropriate to the youths' needs and interests. Children with chronic diseases, risk factors for chronic diseases, and physical and cognitive disabilities have special physical activity needs. Obese children and adolescents, for example, should be referred to a physical activity and nutrition program for overweight young people.

Advocate for school and community physical activity instruction and programs that meet the needs of young people.

To help create physical and social environments that encourage physical activity, health-care providers should advocate for physical education curricula, extracurricular activities, and community sports and recreation programs that emphasize safe, enjoyable lifetime physical activities. Physicians, school nurses, and other health-care professionals can support physical activity among children and adolescents by becoming involved in school and community physical activity initiatives. Within schools many nurses are already involved in joint activities or projects with physical education and health education teachers. Physicians can volunteer to serve as advisors to schools and other community organizations that provide physical activity instruction and programs to young people. Health-care providers should advocate that coaches be trained to make certain that young people compete safely and thrive physically, emotionally, and socially. Health-care providers also should encourage parents to be role models for their children, plan physical activities that involve the whole family, and discuss with their children the value of healthy behaviors such as physical activity.

9 COMMUNITY PROGRAMS

Provide a range of developmentally appropriate community sports and recreation programs that are attractive to all young people.

Most physical activity among children and adolescents occurs outside the school setting. Thus, community sports and recreation programs are integral to promoting physical activity among young people. These community programs can complement the efforts of schools by providing children and adolescents opportunities to engage in the types and levels of physical activity that may not be offered in school. Community sports and recreation programs also provide an avenue for reaching out-of-school young people.

Provide a diversity of developmentally appropriate community sports and recreation programs for all young people.

Young people become involved in structured physical activity programs for various reasons: to develop competence, to build social relationships, to enhance fitness, and to have fun. However, adolescents' participation in community sports and recreation programs declines with age. Many young people drop out of these programs because the activities are not fun, are too competitive, or demand too much time. Because definitions of fun and success vary with each person's age, sex, and skill level, community sports and recreation programs should assess and try to meet the needs and interests of all young people. These programs should also try to match the skill level of the participants with challenges that encourage skill development and fun and to develop programs that are not based exclusively on winning.

Provide access to community sports and recreation programs for young people.

In most communities, physical activity programs for young people exist, but these opportunities often require transportation, fees, or special equipment. These limitations often discourage children and adolescents from low-income families from participating. Communities should ensure that all young people, irrespective of their family's income, have access to these programs. For example, community sports and recreation programs can collaborate with schools and other community organizations such as places of worship to provide transportation to these programs. Communities can also ask businesses to sponsor youth physical activity programs and to provide children and adolescents from low-income families with appropriate equipment, clothing, and footwear for participation in physical activity.

10 EVALUATION

Regularly evaluate school and community physical activity instruction, programs, and facilities.

Evaluation can be used to assess and improve physical activity policies, spaces and facilities, instruction, programs, personnel training, health services, and student achievement. All groups involved in and affected by school and community programs to promote lifelong physical activity among young people should have the opportunity to contribute to evaluation. Valid evaluations may increase support for and involvement in these programs by students, parents, teachers, and other school and community personnel.

Evaluate the implementation and quality of physical activity policies, curricula, instruction, programs, and personnel training.

Evaluation is useful for gaining insight into the implementation and quality of physical activity policies, physical activity spaces and facilities, physical education and health education curricula and instruction, extracurricular and community sports and recreation programs, and preservice and in-service training programs for personnel. The Child and Adolescent Trial for Cardiovascular Health (CATCH) has developed a model that can be used to assess the quantity and quality of physical education instruction, lesson content, fidelity of curriculum implementation, and opportunities for other physical activity. National competency frameworks, including *National Standards for Athletic Coaches: Quality Coaches, Quality Sports; National Standards for Beginning Physical Education Teachers; A Guide for the Development of Competency-Based Curricula for Entry Level Health Educators;* and *Health Instruction Responsibilities and Competencies for Elementary (K–6) Classroom Teachers* can be used to assess the competencies of coaches, entry-level physical education and health education teachers, and elementary school teachers, in addition to the quality of professional training programs for these people. Parents and guardians can use the checklist developed by the National Association for Sport and Physical Education to evaluate the quality of sports and physical activity programs for their children. Other guidelines exist to assess the provision of health services for children and adolescents and the safety of playgrounds.

Measure students' attainment of physical activity knowledge, achievement of motor and behavioral skills, and adoption of healthy behaviors.

Measuring students' achievement in physical education requires a comprehensive assessment of their knowledge, motor and behavioral skills, and behavior related to physical activity. Measuring students' achievement in health education requires an assessment of their knowledge, behavioral skills, and behaviors. *Moving Into the Future: National Standards for Physical Education* and *National Health Education Standards: Achieving Health Literacy* describe what students should know and be able to do as a result of comprehensive physical education and health education programs. Students' achievement may be measured using paper-and-pencil tests that assess knowledge and performance tests that assess motor and behavioral skills. Portfolios of students' work that reflect their knowledge, motor and behavioral skills, and progress toward personal physical activity goals are appropriate for assessing students' achievement. Although fitness testing is a common component of many school physical education programs, the test results should not be used to assign report card grades or assess program effectiveness.

CONCLUSION

School and community programs that promote regular physical activity among young people could be among the most effective strategies for reducing the public health burden of chronic diseases associated with sedentary lifestyles. Programs that provide students with the knowledge, attitudes, motor skills, behavioral skills, and confidence to participate in physical activity may establish active lifestyles among young people that

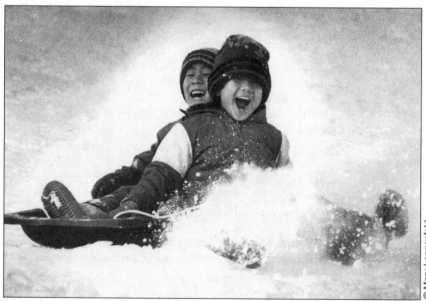

© Mary Langenfeld

Young people should be taught that physical activity is important and that it is fun.

continue into and throughout their adult lives. These programs can promote physical activity by establishing physical activity policies; providing physical and social environments that enable safe and enjoyable participation in physical activity; implementing planned and sequential physical education and health education curricula and instruction from kindergarten through 12th grade; providing extracurricular physical activity programs; including parents and guardians in physical activity instruction and programs; providing personnel training in methods to effectively promote physical activity; providing health services that encourage and support physical activity; providing community-based sports and recreation programs; and evaluating school and community physical activity instruction, programs, and facilities.

GUIDELINES HANDOUTS

As you can see from the guidelines, many members of the community can help promote more and better physical activity opportunities for young people. Two handouts have been included here to assist you in spreading the word. The first is applicable to the public, school staff, and those involved in community physical activity. The second speaks to the staff of institutions of higher education, with specific recommendations for them.

PROMOTING LIFELONG PHYSICAL ACTIVITY AMONG YOUNG PEOPLE

How You Can Help

Everyone can make a difference in young people's lives by helping them include physical activity in their daily routines. If you are a parent, guardian, student, teacher, athletic coach, school administrator or board member, community sports and recreation program coordinator, or anyone else who cares about the health of young people, here are some steps you can take.

Everyone Can

- advocate for convenient, safe, and adequate places for young people to play and take part in physical activity programs;
- encourage school administrators and board members to support daily physical education and other school programs that promote lifelong physical activity, not just competitive sports;
- set a good example by being physically active, making healthy eating choices, and not smoking;

- tell young people about sports and recreation programs in their community; and
- discourage the use of physical activity as a punishment.

Parents or Guardians Can

- encourage your children to be physically active;
- learn what your children want from physical activity programs and help them choose appropriate activities;
- volunteer to help your children's sports teams and recreation programs;
- play and be physically active with your children; and
- teach your children safety rules and make sure that they have the clothing and equipment needed to participate safely in physical activity.

Students Can

- set goals for increasing your physical activity and monitor your progress;
- encourage friends and family members to be physically active;
- use protective clothing and proper equipment to prevent injuries and illnesses;
- encourage the student council to advocate for physical education classes and after-school programs that are attractive to all students; and
- take elective courses in health and physical education.

Teachers and Coaches Can

- use curricula that follow CDC's *Guidelines for School and Community Programs to Promote Lifelong Physical Activity Among Young People* and the national standards for physical education and health education;
- keep students moving during physical education classes;
- ensure that young people know safety rules and use appropriate protective clothing and equipment;
- emphasize activity and enjoyment over competition;
- help students become competent in many motor and behavioral skills;
- involve families and community organizations in physical activity programs; and
- refrain from using physical activity, such as doing push-ups or running laps, as punishment.

School Administrators and Board Members Can

- require health education and daily physical education for students in grades K through 12;
- ensure that physical education and extracurricular programs offer lifelong activities such as walking and dancing;
- provide time during the day, such as recess, for unstructured physical activity such as walking or jumping rope;

- hire physical activity specialists and qualified coaches;
- ensure that school facilities are clean, safe, and open to students during nonschool hours and vacations;
- provide health promotion programs for faculty and staff; and
- provide teachers with in-service training in physical activity promotion.

Community Sports and Recreation Program Coordinators Can

- provide a mix of competitive team sports and noncompetitive, lifelong fitness and recreation activities;
- increase the availability of parks, public swimming pools, hiking and biking trails, and other places for physical activity;
- ensure that physical facilities meet or exceed safety standards;
- ensure that coaches have appropriate coaching competencies; and
- work with schools, businesses, and community groups to ensure that low-income young people have transportation and appropriate equipment for physical activity programs.

PROMOTING LIFELONG PHYSICAL ACTIVITY AMONG YOUNG PEOPLE

How Staffs of Institutions of Higher Education Can Help

You play an important role in preparing education, health, and recreation professionals to help young people establish lifelong involvement in physical activity. In addition, your research efforts can strengthen our knowledge of the most effective strategies for promoting physical activity among young people. Here are some steps you can take to make a difference in young people's lives.

- Use the Centers for Disease Control and Prevention's physical activity guidelines to provide teachers, coaches, administrators, and other school personnel with preservice and in-service training that enables them to promote enjoyable, lifelong physical activity among young people.
- Ensure that physical education teachers and coaches have the competencies specified by the National Association for Sport and Physical Education.
- Place more emphasis on behavioral science in curricula used for training physical education teachers; include courses on methods for producing behavioral change at both the individual and community levels.
- Train teachers to use active learning strategies, build students' confidence in their ability to engage in lifetime physical activity, and keep students moving for most of physical education class time.

- Train school and community personnel to involve parents and the community in physical activity programs for young people.
- Implement summer school courses, short courses, and workshops to instruct physical education and health education teachers on using the CDC physical activity guidelines.
- Build class projects around the CDC physical activity guidelines to increase familiarity with them.
- Conduct research on physical activity, physical education, and health education.
- Encourage colleagues and students to conduct research on the efficacy and effectiveness of different strategies for implementing the recommendations in the guidelines.
- Use the guidelines to assess the physical activity needs of schools and communities.
- Work with schools to evaluate physical education programs and inform school boards about the results.
- Provide the news media with data on the health benefits of physical activity for young people and the effects of well-designed physical education programs.
- Make data-based presentations to school boards about the importance of physical activity for young people, the need for quality physical education, and the value of community partnerships.
- Help student interns develop links between schools and community programs.

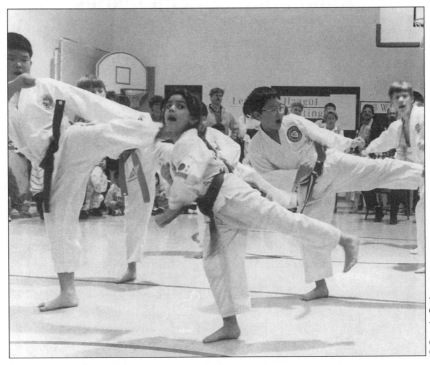

Part II

Success Stories

© Connie Springer

Part II contains 20 stories of programs across the country that have implemented specific CDC guidelines recommendations. In most cases these programs have not been subjected to rigorous evaluation; they have, however, met many of the needs of the local school and community.

To tie these programs to the corresponding guidelines, we have outlined below the main guideline recommendations and followed each recommendation with a list of the numbers of the related stories (in bold). For example, the guideline "Provide health promotion programs for school faculty and staff" is followed by the numbers **2, 5, 9**, and **17**. This means implementation of this guideline is illustrated by the stories in 2, 5, 9, and 17.

Main Points of Guidelines

1 POLICY

Establish policies that promote enjoyable, lifelong physical activity among young people.

- Require comprehensive, daily physical education for students in kindergarten through grade 12. **1, 14**
- Require comprehensive health education for students in kindergarten through grade 12.
- Require that adequate resources, including budget and facilities, be committed for physical activity instruction and programs. **1, 2, 3, 5, 7, 14**
- Require the hiring of physical education specialists to teach physical education in kindergarten through grade 12, elementary school teachers trained to teach health education, health education specialists to teach health education in middle and senior high schools, and qualified people to direct school and community physical activity programs and to coach young people in sports and recreation programs. **3**
- Require that physical activity instruction and programs meet the needs and interests of all students. **1, 7, 17**

2 ENVIRONMENT

Provide physical and social environments that encourage and enable safe and enjoyable physical activity.

- Provide access to safe spaces and facilities for physical activity in the school and the community. **1, 2, 3, 5, 6, 12, 13, 14, 18**

- Establish and enforce measures to prevent physical activity–related injuries and illnesses. **2**
- Provide time within the school day for unstructured physical activity. **8**
- Discourage the use or withholding of physical activity as punishment.
- Provide health promotion programs for school faculty and staff. **3, 4, 6, 14**

3 PHYSICAL EDUCATION

Implement physical education curricula and instruction that emphasize enjoyable participation in physical activity and that help students develop the knowledge, attitudes, motor skills, behavioral skills, and confidence needed to adopt and maintain physically active lifestyles.

- Provide planned and sequential physical education curricula from kindergarten through grade 12 that promote enjoyable, lifelong physical activity. **1, 3, 8**
- Use physical education curricula consistent with the national standards for physical education. **8**
- Use active learning strategies and emphasize enjoyable participation in physical education class. **1, 7, 10, 11, 12, 13, 19**
- Develop students' knowledge of and positive attitudes toward physical activity. **1, 3, 7, 8, 9, 10, 11, 12, 13, 14, 19, 20**
- Develop students' mastery of and confidence in motor and behavioral skills for participating in physical activity. **1, 3, 5, 7, 8, 9, 10, 11, 12, 13, 16, 19, 20**
- Provide a substantial percentage of each student's recommended weekly amount of physical activity in physical education classes. **1, 7, 9, 11, 12**
- Promote participation in enjoyable physical activity in the school, community, and home. **1, 3, 7, 10, 11, 12, 13, 14, 16, 19, 20**

4 HEALTH EDUCATION

Implement health education curricula and instruction that help students develop the knowledge, attitudes, behavioral skills, and confidence needed to adopt and maintain physically active lifestyles.

- Provide planned and sequential health education curricula from kindergarten through grade 12 that promote lifelong participation in physical activity.

- Use health education curricula consistent with the national standards for health education.
- Promote collaboration among physical education, health education, and classroom teachers as well as teachers in related disciplines who plan and implement physical activity instruction. **4, 11, 20**
- Use active learning strategies to emphasize enjoyable participation in physical activity in the school, community, and home. **4, 11, 16, 19, 20**
- Develop students' knowledge of and positive attitudes toward healthy behaviors, particularly physical activity. **4, 6, 13, 14, 16, 19, 20**
- Develop students' mastery of and confidence in the behavioral skills needed to adopt and maintain a healthy lifestyle that includes regular physical activity. **4, 11, 16, 19, 20**

5 EXTRACURRICULAR ACTIVITES

Provide extracurricular physical activity programs that meet the needs and interests of all students.

- Provide a diversity of developmentally appropriate competitive and noncompetitive physical activity programs for all students. **6, 12, 17, 18**
- Link students to community physical activity programs, and use community resources to support extracurricular physical activity programs. **7, 11, 16, 18**

6 PARENTAL INVOLVEMENT

Include parents and guardians in physical activity instruction and in extracurricular and community physical activity programs, and encourage them to support their children's participation in enjoyable physical activities.

- Encourage parents to advocate for quality physical activity instruction and programs for their children.
- Encourage parents to support their children's participation in appropriate, enjoyable physical activities. **4, 6, 7, 11, 13, 14, 16, 19, 20**
- Encourage parents to be physically active role models and to plan and participate in family activities that include physical activity. **4, 7, 11, 13, 14, 19, 20**

7   PERSONNEL TRAINING

Provide training for education, coaching, recreation, health- care, and other school and community personnel that imparts the knowledge and skills needed to effectively promote enjoyable, lifelong physical activity among young people.

- Train teachers to deliver physical education that provides a substantial percentage of each student's recommended weekly amount of physical activity. **7**
- Train teachers to use active learning strategies needed to develop students' knowledge about, attitudes toward, skills in, and confidence in engaging in physical activity. **7, 8, 9, 13, 16, 19**
- Train school and community personnel how to create psychosocial environments that enable young people to enjoy physical activity instruction and programs. **4, 9**
- Train school and community personnel how to involve parents and the community in physical activity instruction and programs. **7**
- Train volunteers who coach sports and recreation programs for young people.

8   HEALTH SERVICES

Assess physical activity patterns among young people, counsel them about physical activity, refer them to appropriate programs, and advocate for physical activity instruction and programs for them.

- Regularly assess the physical activity patterns of young people, reinforce physical activity among active young people, counsel inactive young people about physical activity, and refer young people to appropriate physical activity programs.
- Advocate for school and community physical activity instruction and programs that meet the needs of young people. **16**

9   COMMUNITY PROGRAMS

Provide a range of developmentally appropriate community sports and recreation programs that are attractive to all young people.

- Provide a diversity of developmentally appropriate community sports and recreation programs for all young people. **15, 18**

- Provide access to community sports and recreation programs for young people. **14**

10 EVALUATION

Regularly evaluate school and community physical activity instruction, programs, and facilities.

- Evaluate the implementation and quality of physical activity policies, curricula, instruction, programs, and personnel training. **8, 14**
- Measure students' attainment of physical activity knowledge, achievement of motor and behavioral skills, and adoption of healthy behaviors. **8, 9, 10, 11, 12, 19**

Clovis High School Program

1

Clovis, California

Cliff Wetzel
Department Chairperson
Physical Education Department
Clovis High School
1055 Fowler Avenue
Clovis, CA 93611-2099
(209) 299-7211

■ Policy
■ Environment
■ Physical Education

Program Objectives

- To offer a diverse four-year physical education curriculum that meets students' interests and provides them with the skills and knowledge to take responsibility for personal health
- To give seniors a chance to experience teaching physical education to elementary school students
- To give community members access to and instruction in physical activity

Program at a Glance

Clovis High School is in a school district in California that has maintained a requirement of four years of high school physical education. For the first two years students follow the standard state core curriculum, but the following two years they can choose from a wide range of electives. The school has helped maintain community support for physical education by opening the school's facilities to community use and offering many adult physical activity courses taught by district instructors.

Clovis is a bedroom community for Fresno, a city of about a half million in central California. Much of the community consists of new housing developments, and many people come to Clovis because of the excellent reputation of the school system. Most students are from a middle-class background, and the student population of 3,000 is about 64 percent white, 20 percent Hispanic, 10 percent Asian, 3 percent African American, and around 1 percent each Native American, Filipino, and Pacific Islander.

The Clovis High School Physical Education Curriculum

Clovis is in the only district in California that still requires high school students to take four years of physical education. This goes back to the philosophy of Dr. Floyd Buchanan, a former superintendent who strongly believed that students should build strong bodies and spirits, as well as minds. He also felt that if students were involved in school-related extracurricular activities, whether they be sports, music, debate, or other special areas, they would feel some attachment to the school and be less likely to drop out or engage in unhealthy behaviors.

After students complete the state-mandated physical education courses in their first two years, they are eligible to sign up for any one of a number of elective courses. Courses offered at Clovis High include the following:

- Introductory dance
- Advanced dance
- Honors dance repertory, which culminates in a three-night dance performance for the community
- Team and individual sports, such as badminton, tennis, volleytennis, volleyball, softball, skiing, bowling, basketball, football, street hockey, soccer, or water polo
- High intensity physical education, which may include wrestling, slow pitch softball, street hockey, basketball, team handball, football, weights, or water polo
- Lifetime sports, which may cover racquet sports, volleyball, skiing, bowling, golf, snorkeling, scuba diving, Frisbee, basketball, or wellness/weight training
- Aerobics class (including aqua aerobics and weight training)

- Strength and conditioning, in which students develop individual total fitness programs
- Sports therapy and fitness technician, a work experience funded by the state that is held off-site
- Cross-age physical education, in which seniors teach physical education to elementary school students

The lifetime sports course is one of the more popular electives. Some of these course activities require special equipment or include field trips to golf courses and bowling alleys, but the school has been inventive in finding ways to keep costs down. For example, for the skiing portion of the course, they have been able to purchase used rental equipment from a local store for use in practicing at school. For the field trip, they have found a skiing resort in Yosemite that gives the students a deal on a one-day trip. The school's principal also offsets some costs and pays for the charter bus for the trip. If any of the students have trouble getting the money to go, the principal usually will subsidize their fees as well.

The newest course to be offered will be an adventure course for seniors. It will meet during the last period of the day so class time can be extended, as many of the activities will take place off campus. Activities will include fishing, outdoor education, canoeing, sailing, cycling, skiing, water sports, a guided canoeing trip that looks at the river environment, and a trip to a ski resort that offers a combination skiing/ecology class.

An additional physical education option was developed to accommodate honor students who were having difficulty fitting physical education into an already crowded schedule. In order to allow students to take extra academic classes and yet meet the four-year physical education requirement, the district developed a Directed Study Program. In this program, students are allowed to participate in physical activity outside of school to meet the physical education requirement. They meet with an advisor once a week to review the activities they've completed.

Cross-Age Physical Education

The most unusual of the electives offered at Clovis is the cross-age physical education course, developed by district curriculum specialist Susan Fugman. Only seniors who meet high academic standards may take this course. These students receive four weeks of training in the California physical education curriculum from a district instructor, then are assigned in pairs to an elementary school classroom in the district. Under the supervision of the classroom teacher, the high school students teach the elementary school children physical education for an hour four days a week. The district instructor rotates from school to school to observe the high school students at work.

The high school students must have their own transportation to the elementary schools. Their hour of teaching is scheduled to either precede lunch or be the last period of the school day, so they don't miss any of their academic classes if they have trouble getting back on time.

This course has worked well for everyone involved—high school students, classroom teachers, and elementary school students. The high school students feel it builds their sense of responsibility and confidence, and they enjoy working with the younger kids. The classroom teachers think that the high school students are good role models for their classes. And the elementary students think working with the high school seniors is fun!

Opening School Facilities to the Community

Clovis High School has excellent physical activity facilities. This is because the school district has been able to pass tax bond initiatives in which the money collected can only be spent on physical education or fine arts facilities. The facilities at the high school include the following:

- Twelve lighted tennis courts
- A new all-weather track
- A swimming pool and diving pool
- Two gymnasiums
- A weight room
- A dance studio
- A wrestling and tumbling room

To pay back the community for its generosity, the school in turn has made its facilities available for community members' use during nonschool hours. District instructors run adult physical education programs such as year-round aquatics or strength training in the evenings. An adult tennis league uses the tennis courts at lunch time. This access to the facilities gives the community a pride of ownership in the school.

Conclusion

The Clovis High School program is a great example of how a program can flourish if the proper foundation is provided and maintained. By first developing a curriculum that met the diverse needs of its students and then working closely with the entire community, Clovis High School has been able to win and keep the support of parents, taxpayers, the school board, and the community at large.

Cliff Wetzel, physical education department chair, says he has met students who left high school five or six years ago who still remember how much fun the skiing classes were—and who are still skiing today. People remember quality educational experiences and will support quality programs as they move into decision-making roles in the community.

Further, the high school has bonded with the community by making its physical activity facilities available to all, promoting community wellness. The physical education program at Clovis High School continues to uphold the standards of a sound body, mind, and spirit.

If you are interested in seeing a list of the course offerings in the Clovis High School curriculum, contact Cliff Wetzel at the address or phone number shown at the beginning of this story.

Changing Class Size Policy in Tennessee

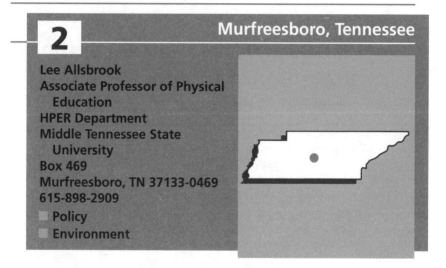

2 **Murfreesboro, Tennessee**

Lee Allsbrook
Associate Professor of Physical
  Education
HPER Department
Middle Tennessee State
  University
Box 469
Murfreesboro, TN 37133-0469
615-898-2909
  ■ Policy
  ■ Environment

Program Objectives

- To end the granting of waivers that allowed for oversized physical education classes in Tennessee schools
- To communicate with the Tennessee State Board of Education about physical education issues

Program at a Glance

Lee Allsbrook, as a representative of the Tennessee Association for Health, Physical Education, Recreation and Dance (TAHPERD), mounted a successful challenge to a proposal to the State Board of Education to continue allowing waivers for physical education classes above recommended class sizes.

Program Background

For many years the Tennessee Board of Education had routinely given local schools waivers for physical education class sizes of as many as 40 to 75 children per class, approximately double the normal class size. In earlier years local schools financed physical education specialists from their own funds; therefore, state board members felt the board should not be the ones to determine class size. The Tennessee AHPERD felt strongly that such large classes weren't good for children's learning or safety.

TAHPERD's Involvement With the State Board of Education

In 1990 the Tennessee AHPERD decided to assign a member to attend each meeting of the State Board of Education, held four to five times a year. This person could observe the proceedings and be available to answer questions from the board related to physical education and health issues.

The person assigned was Lee Allsbrook, a professor at Middle Tennessee State University and an elementary physical education specialist. Lee had, in fact, already been attending state board meetings for some years and was known by the board members.

Issue of Class Size

For some time Lee had spoken at state board meetings against granting waivers for larger-than-recommended classes, commonly referred to as double classes. His first approach was to tell board members that large classes worked against children's fitness. It meant children spent much time standing in line and waiting for a turn or for equipment. The board rejected this idea, saying that the same could be said for any subject: the smaller the class size, the better the children would become at the subject.

The next approach was to say that children in large classes couldn't learn physical skills as well because they received little or no individual attention and didn't get enough opportunities to practice the skills. This also was rejected by the board for much the same reasons as the first approach.

RESISTANCE FROM CLASSROOM TEACHERS

Lee went to the state teachers' association to ask for its help. However, he found that some classroom teachers were opposed to smaller physical education classes because they were afraid that they would lose some of the planning time they had when students were in physical education class. They proposed that Lee not ask for single classes until they could get assurances that funding for enough physical education specialists to handle the additional smaller classes was in place, but Lee felt that would take too long. Although Lee was viewed favorably by the teachers' association because he had been the president of several local teachers' associations and had demonstrated his interest in the whole school curriculum, he ultimately was opposed by the state teachers' association at a state board meeting.

PHYSICAL EDUCATION SPECIALISTS' CONCERNS

Surprisingly enough, even some physical education specialists were opposed to having single classes. Many had spent their whole teaching careers working with oversized classes, and they had developed good management systems for handling them. They also were concerned that breaking up large classes into smaller ones would mean teaching twice as many classes.

Another concern for both physical education specialists and principals was where the additional classes would be held. Many schools had little space available for physical education classes. In fact, one state board member brought up the idea that the money for a new gym for each school should be found before the change was made. Again, Lee felt that this would take too long, and he suggested to the board that teachers could find ways to adapt to the change and that local communities would respond to the need for more space. If making the change was a mistake, Lee said, the board always could reverse the decision.

Proposal for Continued Class Size Waivers

In October 1991 the State Board of Education agenda included a proposal to continue granting waivers for physical education classes to exceed recommended class sizes. This time Lee spoke against it on the basis of the danger to children and the schools' liability. In fact, some classroom teachers testified that they had had to treat several children who had been injured during oversized physical education classes.

After that meeting a reporter who had covered it decided to do a story on the safety of double classes. He visited a Nashville elementary school to observe an oversized class and talk with the teachers. One of the teachers interviewed said that teaching oversized classes meant she had to give higher priority to supervising children than to teaching the curriculum. Afterward the reporter went to the public records to find out how many children had been injured during such classes and found a startling number of injuries. The subsequent article won over many board members.

On the day of the vote on the proposal in November 1990, the board member who put the issue up for a vote talked about what had made him decide against waivers. He said that just recently he had taken his six-year-old daughter and five of her friends to a children's pizza parlor and had had a hard time keeping them under control in that setting. Based on that experience, he found it hard to believe that children weren't at risk in a physical education class that might contain up to ten times more children. The one student member of the state board also happened to be a former student from Lee's single-class physical education program. Without any prompting from Lee, he stated that he found it hard to believe that the state allowed double classes.

The vote against allowing waivers to local schools was unanimous. Because the change in class size was made in the middle of the school year, some of the additional classes were taken over by classroom teachers. However, by a year or two later, most schools had found the money so classes were taught by elementary physical education specialists.

Observations on Working With the State Board of Education

From this and other experiences with the State Board of Education, Lee has drawn a number of conclusions on how to best approach and work with board members.

• Board members care about the welfare of school children and want to do what's right for students. However, they are bombarded with requests from both inside and outside the school, hearing from many people on many issues. Therefore, even though you are a representative of a group concerned about an issue, you should not take on an adversarial role.

• You don't have to be a polished speaker to speak before the board. In fact, if the presentation is too polished and is designed only to promote your point of view, board members may wonder if they can get straight answers from you. On the other hand, board members may ask you hard questions and expect quick answers. Therefore, it is important to practice and brainstorm possible questions and good answers before presenting.

- Board members will examine your motivations when you speak before them. If you are at meetings frequently, board members will talk to you to find out why you are there and if you are a paid lobbyist. To inspire board members' confidence in you, you need to attend board meetings regularly and show your concern for *all* aspects of the school curriculum, not just the one of interest to you. Many people come to one meeting to advocate their particular point of view and then leave as soon as discussion of that point is over.

- Many people go to board meetings only to try to "win" for their viewpoint. They are unwilling to compromise. It's better to be flexible in your views. If the board members hear merit in several viewpoints on the same issue, they will set up meetings on the issue with advocates to try to reach a stand that will include the best parts of each. Know in advance how much you are willing to compromise.

- It's important to persevere in your attempt to change policy. Try different arguments and don't be afraid to involve the media.

Conclusion

Regular attendance at state board of education meetings is a vital step in attempting to change policy. In Tennessee a combination of one person's persistence and sound strategic planning by TAHPERD proved to be successful.

Lincoln County Schools Program

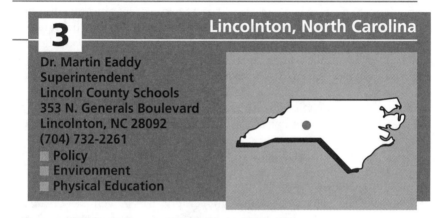

3

Lincolnton, North Carolina

Dr. Martin Eaddy
Superintendent
Lincoln County Schools
353 N. Generals Boulevard
Lincolnton, NC 28092
(704) 732-2261
▪ Policy
▪ Environment
▪ Physical Education

Program Objectives

- To develop lifelong physical activity skills
- To teach students how physical activity contributes to lifelong health
- To teach stress management techniques to school staff

Program at a Glance

In 1986 a retired businessman who was a fitness enthusiast lobbied for sweeping changes to the Lincoln County School District's physical education program; the result has been improved and enriched physical education at all grade levels. Several district schools have been chosen by the state as demonstration schools for physical education, and special additions have been made to the program. These include a ropes course for each middle school and a new aerobics/weight lifting facility for high school students that also is available to school and community agency staff.

Program Background

The Lincoln County School District includes 9,800 students and 700 certified staff. It is a rural district located between Charlotte, North Carolina, and the edges of the Blue Ridge Mountains. Manufacturing, service, and farming are the mainstays of the local economy.

The Beginning of Changes in the District

Today Lincoln County School District has an exceptional physical education program, but it might not be that way had it not been for the efforts of one man, Caldwell Nixon. In 1986, Caldwell was a retired businessman who was physically active and a winner of national medals for running and walking in the Senior Olympics. He felt strongly that children need quality physical education to stay active throughout life, and he brought his concerns directly to Lincoln County Schools Superintendent Dr. Martin Eaddy. Responding to the challenge, Martin and the school board decided to hire enough physical education specialists for one to be available at each school in the district. This was paid for by extra funding from the state for teachers in speciality areas. They also asked state-funded consultants to help them completely rework the district's curriculum.

The new elementary school curriculum emphasizes movement education, with a focus on coordination, balance, strength, and movement fun. The content of physical education classes is coordinated with what children learn in health education. At the middle school level, physical education courses focus on recreational activities and team sports. Recreational businesses and community agencies have helped support off-site physical education activities, such as bowling, swimming, or golf, held during the school day by charging students lower rates for use of their facilities.

One of the goals of the curriculum is for all children to meet state standards for physical education. All children also participate in the President's Challenge Physical Fitness Program test.

Program Additions

With the development of a sound physical education program came several additions that enriched the program.

ROPES COURSES

Each of the district's three middle schools has installed ropes courses, multilevel pieces of equipment made of rope, wire, or wood that pose individual and group challenges. By solving the challenges, course participants build team skills, commitment, healthy attitudes, and higher self-esteem.

These courses were developed by the district's Alcohol and Drug Defense Coordinator, with support from a federal grant and donations from local businesses.

In return for this support, businesses are allowed to use the ropes courses twice a year to train their management teams. They pay a fee for this privilege, and district instructors are on hand to assist them.

FITNESS CENTER

One of the district's high schools recently created a new fitness center. This project started with a football coach's desire for a weight lifting center for his team. He first talked the district into giving him an old, unused automotive mechanics facility as space for the center. He then went to local businesses that had supported school team sports in the past and asked for donations to obtain weight equipment. This resulted in being able to obtain about $9,000 worth of equipment.

The center became part of the general physical education curriculum. Physical education students set individual goals and can then use the equipment in the center to achieve those goals within a given time period. Once the center was open, staff started to get interested. They wanted to use the weight machines, too, and suggested—and got—aerobic machines.

Today the center is available not only to school students and staff, but also to community agencies that need such a facility. This includes the police and sheriff's departments and the fire department. Physical education instructors volunteer to keep the facility open three nights a week for school staff and community agency members to use at no charge.

Conclusion

This is a case in which an initial push from a concerned citizen, Caldwell Nixon, was the impetus for a whole series of improvements in the school district's physical education program through a combination of seeking available state education funds and community fundraising. Physical education focused on movement education and lifetime activities, and was coordinated with the school health education program. Demonstration schools were developed, providing the district's physical education teachers with resources for improving their classes.

The story also illustrates how communities and schools can form partnerships to improve and share physical education facilities. The ropes courses were added with partial funding from the local businesses, and business owners in turn have been given the opportunity to use the facilities for their own employees. The new fitness center equipment also was paid for by local businesses, and the school allows local police and fire department members to use the facility.

Wellness Initiatives in Escambia County Schools

4

Escambia County, Florida

Manny Harageones
Specialist, Physical Education,
  Health and Wellness
Escambia County School District
30 East Texar Drive
Pensacola, FL 32503
904-469-5464
  Environment
  Health Education
  Parental Involvement
  Personnel Training

Program Objectives

- To incorporate wellness throughout the school curriculum and environment
- To help all employees and students develop healthy lifestyles
- To form partnerships with community health organizations in order to promote wellness for staff and students
- To involve parents in developing student and family wellness

Program at a Glance

Escambia County Schools have a number of district- and school-level wellness initiatives serving district and school staff and students. In the future, the program will also serve parents.

Program Background

Escambia County is located on the west coast of northern Florida. It contains both rural and urban schools and many beach communities. A Navy base is located in Pensacola, the largest city in the county. The school district serves 45,000 children and has 5,500 employees.

History of the Initiatives

After participating in a 1994 Florida Department of Education wellness workshop, Escambia County education officials chose to develop both district-level and school-level wellness initiatives. All initiatives are developed and implemented by wellness teams that consist of many different types of people. Physical education teachers often take a leadership role, although school administrators, school nurses, cafeteria managers, guidance counselors, building janitors, teachers, parents, and other school and community members are also included.

District-Level Initiatives

The district's wellness initiatives are included in its applied strategic plan, which ensures the visibility of the initiatives and makes them eligible for funding. The first initiative was to develop a wellness program for district office employees. This was done in the belief that district staff could not ask schools to do something they were not willing to do themselves. Both district offices set up wellness teams, whose first activity was conducting a survey to identify employees' needs and interests. Employees' responses then were used to develop program activities such as the following:

- Monthly brown-bag lunch seminars
- A monthly wellness newsletter (sponsored by a community hospital)
- Indoor and outdoor walking paths
- Exercise classes after work
- Wellness bulletin boards
- An annual wellness fair (sponsored by all three community hospitals)
- Special events such as challenge and fun walks

The second initiative was forming wellness partnerships with community organizations. The three hospitals in the area have assisted the schools by sponsoring wellness fairs and offering speakers on health topics. Other health-related organizations such as the American Cancer Society, American Diabetes Association, American Heart Association, American Lung Association, and American Red Cross have provided schools with materials and training. The district has also negotiated with local fitness facilities to obtain special corporate rates for district employees.

A third initiative is the Parent Distance Learning Project, which is creating a series of 15-minute videos that show parents how they can serve as wellness role models for their children. Each video will focus on a different

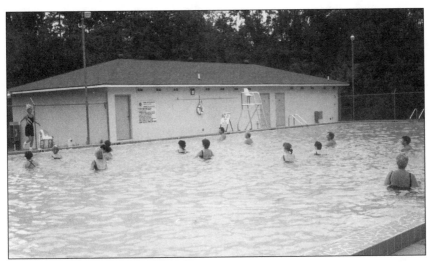

Exercise classes after work for district employees were part of a wellness program initiated by the first district-level initiative.

wellness topic. Copies of the videos will be made available to all schools for presentation at meetings, and the videos will be shown on the local cable television public access channel.

School-Level Initiatives

Longleaf Elementary School's pilot wellness program has moved from an initial emphasis on employees into activities for students. A three-day student wellness fair is held annually incorporating traditional fitness assessment with other types of health assessments, such as hearing and vision. Each assessment is done at a separate station, and students receive feedback at each one. Then, with the help of wellness team members and classroom teachers, each child develops an individual wellness plan (IWP). For very young children, goals are kept few and simple, such as "Eat more vegetables" and "Go for a walk with Mom or Dad once a week." Older students might create measurable goals for each fitness component and other wellness areas.

One year, the school had the entire fifth grade put on a play about wellness. After the play a physician spoke to students and parents about the importance of wellness. Then the children and their parents met with members of the school wellness team and classroom teachers to work out a summer family wellness plan (FWP). Since that time, efforts to help families develop a summer family wellness plan have become an annual event.

Currently, 90% of the schools in the district are developing their own wellness programs. They start by sending wellness teams to a district-sponsored four-day workshop.

The schools that already have wellness programs generate an annual report entitled "Successful Approaches to Wellness," which describes school-level wellness activities. (Copies are available by contacting Manny Harageones. A small fee may be charged to cover copying and shipping.)

Preliminary Program Results

Although the wellness program at Longleaf Elementary School is only three years old, it already has drawn attention and praise. The local school board has awarded the school its Risk Taker Award. The school also has received the Professional Recognition Award from the Florida Alliance for Health, Physical Education, Recreation, Dance and Driver Education (FAHPERD), the Model Physical Fitness School Award from the Florida Governor's Council on Physical Fitness and Sports, and the Little Red Schoolhouse Award from the Florida Elementary School Principals Association. Team members have been invited to talk at national, state, and district meetings.

The district's 49 other wellness schools have developed and implemented many wellness activities for both staff and students that are an integral part of their school improvement efforts. The success of these efforts can be attributed to the wellness team concept of professionals working together to meet the health needs of staff and students.

Conclusion

The Escambia County Schools seem to be well on their way to creating comprehensive wellness programs throughout the district. They began by educating district personnel and getting them to buy into wellness, then moved to activities teachers provided for students. Now, as the schools gain parent support for wellness through individual student and family wellness plans and parent training videos and through community support from school partnerships with health organizations, students will receive a consistent message about the importance of taking responsibility for their own health. The consistent message in the schools and community provides an environment conducive to physical activity and healthful living.

Forest High Campus
SELF Center

5   **Ocala, Florida**

Cindy Repp and Debbie Gallaway
Physical Educators
Forest High School
1416 Southeast Fort King Street
Ocala, FL 34471
352-629-8711
■ Policy
■ Environment
■ Physical Education

Program Objectives

- To create a fitness center where high school students can learn about and practice personal fitness programs
- To make the center available for all students and staff for exercise after school

Program at a Glance

Frustrated by an increasing lack of space for physical education, physical education teachers Cindy Repp and Debbie Gallaway decided that their school needed a fitness center. With the support of their administrators, they went to the community to get the funding needed to purchase equipment. The fitness center is now an integral part of their physical education classes, and they plan to promote it as a facility for after-class use as well.

Program Background

Ocala is a city of 100,000 in north central Florida, about 90 miles from Orlando. Forest High School has 2,000 students, a mix of African Americans, whites, and Hispanics. Students come from a wide range of socioeconomic levels.

The Need for a Fitness Center

Forest High School is located in the middle of a residential district bordered by a historic district, making needed expansion impossible. Yet its student population continues to grow. In September 1994 two physical education teachers, Cindy Repp and Debbie Gallaway, got tired of trying to teach four classes on one field or, when it was rainy, in one gym. The parking lot was the running track, and the basketball and tennis courts had been lost to classroom expansion. They decided that one answer would be to create a school fitness center.

Having a fitness center, with cardiovascular and weight-lifting equipment, would help their students get fit and develop lifetime physical activity skills. Since no state or county funding was available for a center, they decided to seek support from the community.

They began by developing a five-year program plan that they presented to their principal, area physical education supervisor, and superintendent. Once the plan was approved, they began to map out what materials and equipment would be necessary to make their dream a reality. Their goal was to open the center in fall 1995.

Getting Help From the Community

Before going out to raise funds, Cindy and Debbie prepared a summary of the reasons the center was needed and what the center program would do for students. They emphasized the need to promote lifelong fitness skills at the high school level, before students became older and had less access to fitness instruction. They chose and priced the equipment for the center by contacting various exercise equipment manufacturers and talking with experts in the field. And they developed a slide presentation for the community.

Cindy and Debbie had to collect $35,000 in donations to make their dream a reality. A bank contributed $2,000, several physicians donated, and one of Ocala's main hospital gave $15,00. The hospital also offered $10,000 grants to each of the five other high schools in the county over a five-year period. Parents, alumni, business leaders, and many others all helped make the fund-raising successful.

The two teachers worked on this project in their free time and all during the summer. If they couldn't schedule meetings during their lunch hours, other teachers would help by covering their classes.

The Fitness Center

Cindy and Debbie persisted in requesting space from the high school for their fitness center, and in April 1995, a 2,500 square foot former construction classroom finally was made available to them. The area physical education supervisor was able to talk the county into refurbishing the room for its new use, and the center was ready in the fall.

The center presently houses 29 pieces of cardiovascular equipment: 20 stationery bikes, two step machines, two treadmills, and five rowing machines. It also includes 20 Nautilus machines loaned to the school by the University of Florida.

Students in the personal fitness and aerobics classes use the fitness center every other day. Because Forest High has a 90-minute block schedule, half of the period can be spent in the classroom learning physical activity and fitness concepts and the other half in the fitness center. While they are in the center, students must spend at least 15 minutes on cardiovascular training, but they then have the option of either continuing their cardiovascular workout or working out on the Nautilus machines.

At the beginning of the semester, Debbie and Cindy take the class through the center and demonstrate how to use each piece of equipment correctly. After that, students are free to choose which cardiovascular training machine they wish to use.

Teachers observe students as they work out, to make sure they are using correct form. Heart rate monitors are available for all students doing cardiovascular training, so Debbie and Cindy can see if students are working out at their training heart rates. Students are told that their objective is to show improvement in their fitness by the end of the semester.

The University of Florida has sent a graduate assistant to conduct research on the results of students' training. She will be pre- and posttesting students for strength, flexibility, and cardiovascular endurance. The collected data will be made available to the Munroe Regional Medical Center and the university.

Future Plans

Forest High students have enjoyed using the fitness center. They know how to use the equipment safely and properly and work out hard during classes. The center gives them the opportunity to choose their own workout program and to try different types of equipment.

One innovation planned for next year is setting up computers and an animated software program for students to use in tracking progress and designing their own physical activity plans. The school already has the software, but more computers are required to meet class needs.

The fitness center has not been heavily used by students after school, perhaps because most students are bussed to school and would have to find alternate transportation home if they stayed to work out. Cindy and Debbie would like the center to be open two hours a day Monday through Thursday. Next year they plan to promote after-school use of the center by talking to students in classes about finding alternative transportation and by distributing newsletters and flyers and giving presentations at school club meetings.

Although all the initial funding of the center is in place, Cindy and Debbie believe they still have to raise money. For one thing, they'd like to have more treadmills and step machines, which are very popular with students. For another, the warranties held on the machines will eventually expire, so funds will be needed for repairs.

Conclusion

Cindy Repp and Debbie Gallaway's determination led them to find a way to not only overcome a space problem, but also to enrich their program offerings. It took much work on their part, as well as a great deal of support from their administrators. The generosity of the community has allowed them to create a facility that better meets students' physical activity interests and needs.

For a packet of information on the Forest High fitness center, contact Debbie or Cindy at the address or phone number shown at the beginning of this story.

Herbert Hoover High School Fitness Center

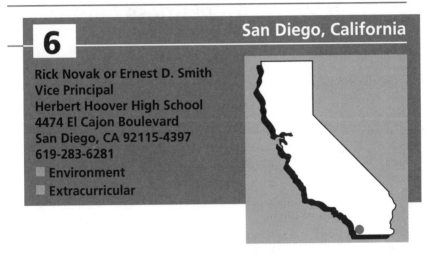

6

San Diego, California

Rick Novak or Ernest D. Smith
Vice Principal
Herbert Hoover High School
4474 El Cajon Boulevard
San Diego, CA 92115-4397
619-283-6281
■ Environment
■ Extracurricular

Program Objectives

- To create a fitness center to serve high school students, staff, and the community

Program at a Glance

Herbert Hoover High School set up a new fitness center with the donation of equipment through the Operation FitKids program in cooperation with the California Governor's Council on Physical Fitness and Sports. The center is staffed by volunteers from the school staff and community, and it serves both students and the surrounding community.

Program Background

Herbert Hoover High School, with an enrollment of 1,920 and growing, has a diverse student body. About 50 percent of students are Hispanic, 21 percent Indo-Chinese, and 20 percent African American; the remainder are other Asian nationalities and white. The community is a starting point for new immigrants; over 50 percent of the senior class last year were foreign-born. Families in the area are not well-off; about 50 percent of Hoover students' families are on some form of welfare or public assistance.

Developing The Fitness Center

The idea for the Herbert Hoover Fitness Center came to the school's athletic director, Ernest P. Smith, on a Friday night in 1994 when he was attending a basketball game at San Diego High. During the game, he took a quick tour of the school's athletic facilities and was amazed when he saw 30 or 40 people working out on a number of shiny new fitness machines—at 6 o'clock on a Friday night, no less. He wanted to know how San Diego High had put together such a state-of-the-art workout facility when his high school had nothing but a small, dingy weight room with a few pieces of worn-out equipment.

It turned out that San Diego High was the recipient of one of the first donations of equipment from Operation FitKids. This national program was founded by Ken Germano, a fitness equipment expert, as a response to a call for assistance from corporate America from the then-chair of the President's Council on Physical Fitness and Sports, Arnold Schwarzenegger. Operation FitKids brought together a consortium of well-known fitness equipment companies, such as Nautilus and StairMaster, to donate hundreds of thousands of dollars' worth of new and used equipment to schools and community organizations nationally. In California, the Governor's Council on Physical Fitness and Sports helps Operation FitKids select sites, and each school that receives such a donation must meet the following criteria:

- The student body must represent various ethnic backgrounds with a large percentage of minorities.
- The economic status of the community should be low- to middle-income.
- The physical education department must be dedicated to a quality physical education curriculum.
- The primary use of the equipment must be designated for coed physical education classes.
- The school must be willing to participate in a preassessment program administered by the Governor's Council.
- The school must establish an after-school fitness club open to all students, faculty, and staff.
- The school must participate in a three-hour in-service/staff development workshop conducted by the staff of the Governor's Council and Operation FitKids.

- The school must assume full responsibility for the maintenance of all Operation FitKids equipment.
- The school must be willing to accommodate a press conference/dedication program.

Ernest wanted to start a similar fitness center in his school, so he applied for a grant from Operation FitKids. His request was rejected at first, because there was already one pilot school in the San Diego area. However, Ernest continued to try to raise support for getting equipment for his school. He contacted the city council, his assembly person, and others in government to request that they send letters of support to the Governor's Council. They did, and after a year of persistent work it paid off—Operation FitKids gave Herbert Hoover High $150,000 worth of cardiovascular and strength-training equipment.

On October 10, 1995, Hoover High held a grand opening ceremony for its fitness center that was attended by well-known fitness experts and government dignitaries. Peter Vidmar, 1984 Olympic gold medalist in gymnastics, gave the keynote address and a gymnastics demonstration.

Fitness Center Facilities, Staffing, and Scheduling

Hoover High's new center is housed in a reconditioned small gym that measures 2,800 square feet. It contains areas for aerobics, free weights, strength training, and cardiovascular exercise. The center has rubber flooring, brand-new mirrors, a sound system, and a security system.

The center is used by six different groups:

- Physical education classes
- Athletic teams
- Staff members
- Fitness club members
- Community members
- School volunteers

A fitness club was formed to allow students and community members to work out during non-school hours. A small fee is asked for membership: $2 a month for students, $3 a month for school alumni, and $5 a month for school staff and community members. Fees go to help with equipment maintenance, which is not covered by the school district. Not too many community members have joined yet, but the school hopes to slowly increase the number of members from outside through increased publicity about the availability of the center to the community.

The fitness center is open six days a week for 10 hours a day. During the school day it's staffed by certified teachers; before school, coaches work with athletes and supervise; after school, volunteers staff the center. These volunteers include both school staff and members of the community, many of whom are personal trainers. The diversity of the volunteers is as great as that of the student body itself.

Ernest finds he spends about five to six hours a week running it. One way he's found to cut down the time it takes is to have accounting students check each day's payment of fees and balance the books. This not only helps him, but also gives the students some real-life experience.

The students are very proud of the new center, and about a quarter of the student population have become paid fitness club members. Only one incident of graffiti has come up during the entire year, and the students immediately turned in the person who did it. The students' only complaint is that the center isn't open long enough!

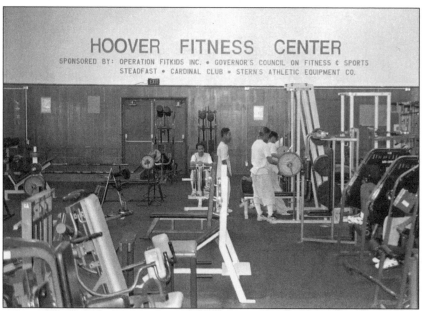

The students at Herbert Hoover High School are very proud of their new fitness center. Although the center is open six days a week, 10 hours a day, students still complain that it is not open long enough.

Future Plans

In the future Ernest wants to try to extend the center's hours, although this might mean that the school would have to begin paying those who staff the center after school (right now volunteers are unpaid). He also would like to get all the teachers in the school who teach relevant curricula, such as science and health, to use the center more in their teaching. Finally, now that the school has obtained appropriate computer hardware and software, he plans to keep a database to see if those who work out in the center also have better attendance and school performance records.

Conclusion

It was Ernest Smith's persistence that made it possible for Hoover High to create a fitness center, one that motivates students to exercise and learn more about healthy lifestyles. It has become a resource that can help the school by improving the physical education program, providing a place for students to work out in their free time, boosting the athletic program, and offering a way to connect with community residents.

Arizona State University/ Mesa Elementary School Cooperative Physical Education Project

7

Mesa, Arizona

Robert Pangrazi
Department of Exercise Science and
  Physical Education
Arizona State University
Tempe, AZ 85287-0701
602-965-3593

- Policy
- Physical Education
- Parent Involvement
- Personnel Training

Program Objectives

- To change the physical education program to emphasize activity and skills development for all children
- To form a partnership between the university and public schools to bring consistency to physical education teaching and teacher training

Program at a Glance

This program has for 23 years helped Mesa elementary school physical education teachers deliver a curriculum in which all children are encouraged to be active. The university does in-service work with district teachers and incorporates the curriculum into its own teacher training.

The program emphasizes parent and community involvement and communication. It has been the combination of quality programming and continual communication with stakeholders that has set the stage for growth—

since the program's inception the number of physical education specialists in the district has slowly but steadily grown from 5 to 70.

Program Background

Mesa is a city of 350,000, with a population that includes many Native
Americans and Mexican Americans. Its school district is the largest in Arizona, including 46 elementary schools that teach 40,000 children.

Program Origins

In 1973 Bob approached the Mesa school district with his new physical
education curriculum. It was designed to reach all children in physical education classes, not just those who are athletically gifted. He felt that there
were plenty of opportunities in the community for highly skilled children
to develop themselves, but that schools must provide opportunities for
children of all skill levels. The curriculum emphasizes constant movement—
no standing in line—and mastery of basic skills.

The district began a pilot project at a single school during the 1974-75
school year. At the beginning there were some hurdles. School maintenance
personnel were unwilling to allow classes to move inside to the cafeteria
when the late summer heat reached over 100 degrees, and teachers were
reluctant to ask for the additional equipment that was necessary for all
children to be active during class. Most of all, many physical education
teachers felt threatened by the new curriculum, which was less sports-oriented than the curricula they had always used. An outside instructor was
brought in to teach the pilot program, but as that program received more
recognition from both within and outside the school system, more and more
teachers became involved. Because the program had clear goals and was
supported by the district, it eventually caught on.

Since that first pilot, the program has branched out to encompass all
Mesa elementary schools. Many other school districts in Arizona have asked
for assistance in learning how to use Mesa's curriculum.

University-School Partnership

In order to ensure that teachers became familiar and comfortable with the
new curriculum, Bob designed and conducted in-service training and cre-

ated a model for enabling Arizona State University physical education students to implement the curriculum.

To do this, Bob met with school principals and physical education supervisors to ask what they wanted to see in a training program. The training was constructed with their input, and a partnership was built between the university and the school district. The district paid for Dr. Pangrazi to present in-service training once a month after school, which teachers were required to attend. School district supervisors could sit in on university teacher training courses to see how the courses were being taught.

Today the Mesa school district has 70 physical education specialists, all trained through Arizona State University. Because these specialists also serve as the cooperating teachers for student teaching at the university, student teachers get a consistent message about how to teach physical education.

The physical education specialists in the Mesa school district all use the same curriculum, and they believe that they are accountable as a group for what they teach. To make sure the curriculum continues to fill teachers' needs, Bob meets with school physical education specialists once a month to discuss the program. They also get together at the end of each school year to evaluate and revise the curriculum to meet new needs.

Parent Involvement

Mesa elementary school physical education teachers try to involve parents and the community in the program. Every school holds an annual Physical Education night, in which teachers demonstrate what goes on in physical education classes. These have been so popular that they have to be held in high school gyms, where there's enough room. Many schools hold family fitness nights, in which parents learn something about fitness and children help them evaluate their own fitness. Family walks and runs also are sponsored.

Teachers regularly send home information about the program. At the start and middle of the year, parents are sent an invitation to come to the school to watch their child's physical education class, and are given easy access to the school on those days.

The teachers' unity and their promotion of the program to the community has given them the clout to get more funding and personnel. For example, each school building has at least $20,000 worth of physical education equipment. The teachers have made sure that each child has the equipment needed to stay active throughout class. Also, during the time that the program has been running, the number of physical education specialists in the district has risen from 5 to 70. At first, money was found for additional physical education specialists by slightly enlarging classroom size to limit the number of classroom teachers required. However, the schools now have budgeted to fund the additional specialist positions.

The Mesa Program Today and Tomorrow

The Mesa program still centers around encouraging less-skilled children, particularly those who are obese. The mile run has been eliminated to avoid embarrassing children, and grades are based on personal best efforts, not comparisons with other children or norms.

As the program has grown, it has also evolved. It recently moved from a focus on fitness and fitness testing to one of encouraging physical activity. It has moved away from sports, especially team sports, toward more life-long activities and a larger variety of activities such as Frisbee golf and orienteering.

A new effort this year will be to get more community organizations involved in providing physical activity for children at all levels of ability. Mesa teachers and university instructors are going to groups such as the YMCA and Boy Scouts to show leaders in those organizations how to run activities for less-skilled children. The idea is to make more opportunities available for all children to be active outside of school.

Conclusion

This program demonstrates how the concerted efforts of a school district and a university can bring about real change in school physical education. The university can develop new programs while the schools in turn can administer the programs and give real-world feedback on curriculum to the university. Teacher training also benefits by offering student teachers a consistent philosophy and structure to follow. Students get the chance to participate in a program that promotes physical activity for everyone. And finally, having a common program and involving parents in the program through parent and family events has helped teachers gain adequate resources for physical education.

Michigan's Exemplary Physical Education Curriculum Project (MI-EPEC)*

8

East Lansing, Michigan

Charles Kuntzleman
Paul Vogel
Michigan's Exemplary Physical
  Education Curriculum Project
40 I.M. Sports Circle
Michigan State University
East Lansing, MI 48824
517-355-5224

■ Physical Education
■ Personnel Training
■ Evaluation

Program Objectives

- To create an exemplary physical education curriculum for use in Michigan's school districts to help students obtain the necessary skills, knowledge, and attitudes to be fit for life
- To develop materials and procedures (including assessment instruments) to be used by those implementing this curriculum

Program at a Glance

Michigan's Exemplary Physical Education Curriculum Project (MI-EPEC) is a state-supported effort to develop, test, and disseminate materials for a model physical education curriculum that will help students meet

---

*Dr. Glenna DeJong, Dr. Paul Vogel, and Dr. Charles Kuntzleman collaborated in the writing of this case study.

carefully selected, specific performance criteria. The curriculum is being developed with the help of physical education specialists and university faculty, and with input from several school districts and physical activity-related organizations.

Program Background

In the early '90s, the governor of Michigan, John Engler, became concerned with the low fitness levels of Michigan youth. To help improve this situation, he charged the newly formed Governor's Council on Physical Fitness with developing materials and procedures to enable schools in Michigan to establish exemplary physical education programs. Michigan's Exemplary Physical Education Curriculum Project (MI-EPEC) was developed to accomplish this task.

Development of the Governor's Council and the Michigan Fitness Foundation

Jan Christensen, a health department official, proposed the Michigan Fitness Foundation as a method of raising both public and private funds to implement the policies and initiatives of the Governor's Council (which cannot receive money directly). Currently the Michigan Fitness Foundation receives about one million dollars a year in state funding, which comes from tobacco taxes. That money is given on a matching funds basis, however, so the Foundation is required to raise additional money to fully fund its programs.

One of the Foundation's four main initiatives is the Michigan Exemplary Physical Education Curriculum Project. Its purpose is to develop a curriculum that will enable those responsible for physical education in Michigan to create exemplary programs.

PROJECT STAFF AND CONSORTIUM

The MI-EPEC project staff, formed in September of 1994, consists of several physical education experts from Michigan State University and the

University of Michigan with specialties in curriculum, instructional design, measurement, evaluation, fitness, and health promotion. In addition, a consortium was formed to advise project staff. Consortium members included representatives of:

- Faculty from seven other universities
- Seven school districts
- State Department of Education
- Governor's Council on Physical Fitness, Health and Sports
- Michigan Parks and Recreation Association
- Michigan Association for Health, Physical Education, Recreation and Dance
- Michigan's Intermediate School Districts

The project team members (staff and consortium members) guide the work of the project and serve as regional coordinators and contacts for physical educators who are involved in the development, implementation, and evaluation of project materials.

SELECTING HIGH-PRIORITY OBJECTIVES

A key part of the development of MI-EPEC was to decide what content should be included in a core curriculum limited to two days a week, 30 minutes a day , which is the amount of time available to most Michigan elementary schools. (As the project continues, materials will be developed for programs that meet more frequently.) The project team obtained ratings of 250 objectives from over 130 physical educators, administrators, and parents representing 18 independent school districts. The team then ranked the objectives on the basis of how highly they were rated on relative importance to an exemplary physical education curriculum. Project members are now developing instructional materials to meet the highest priority program objectives.

As an example, some of the objectives that were identified as high priority for grades K–2 include the following:

- Physical fitness: improving aerobic capacity, building hip/low back flexibility
- Motor skills: running, skipping, throwing, catching
- Cognitive understanding: identifying body parts, actions, and planes; knowing the effects of physical activity
- Personal/social attitudes: following directions, cooperating, giving best effort

DEVELOPING INSTRUCTIONAL MATERIALS

The project members plan to develop instructional resource materials (IRM) for each high-priority objective. Each IRM will include the following information:

- A rationale for the objective
- Program and instructional objectives, including illustrated visual analyses and common performance errors
- Teaching/learning progressions
- Assessment activities, including student evaluation scoresheets
- Instructional activities for each step in the progression
- Ideas for use in the classroom
- Ideas for use during recess, lunch, or after school
- Ideas for homework
- References and resources

Teachers can use the IRMs to develop lessons and instructional strategies. The project staff is using the IRMs to develop lessons, by grade level, for use in various contexts (one-day through five-days-a-week programs). These lessons will help new teachers and teachers who are overloaded to use the information included in the IRMs with less preparation time.

Evaluation of project materials is a high priority for the MI-EPEC team. Consortium members and other content experts are reviewing and revising the first drafts of the IRMs in accordance with specific criteria drawn from the literature. Lessons developed from the IRMs have already been implemented and evaluated by 123 teachers for their feasibility, clarity, quality, appropriateness of assigned time, developmental appropriateness, and perceived effect on student achievement of lesson objectives.

Currently the K–2 lessons are being finalized for publication and dissemination. Work will then shift to grades 3–5 (anticipated completion in summer 1998) and the secondary grade level materials.

DISSEMINATING THE MI-EPEC MATERIALS

To date, the project team has conducted seven workshops that have introduced MI-EPEC materials to over 500 teachers and administrators, emphasizing the need for physical education to make a positive difference in children's lives.

The project team will begin disseminating the K–2 lessons in early 1998 and the grades 3–5 materials shortly thereafter. Those districts adopting the materials must send teachers to an in-service session on how to use the MI-EPEC materials most effectively.

MI-EPEC is expected to become self-sustaining, so that sales of project materials will support future revisions and dissemination. This expectation helped lead to start-up funding from the state legislature.

The project's plans include developing assessment protocols based on the curriculum objectives. Status and progress on high-priority objectives can then be summarized for individual students, classrooms, buildings, and districts. The testing program is to be linked to an eight-level exemplary awards ladder that is offered to schools by the Governor's Council. The first four levels involve completing exemplary programmatic actions, and the second four levels require documentation of student outcomes. The project team recently obtained money to initiate the test development process.

Conclusion

The MI-EPEC project team is committed to providing Michigan schools with a carefully planned curriculum with flexible implementation alternatives. Appropriate use of the materials should help students develop knowledge, skills, and attitudes necessary for lifelong participation in physical activity. Careful evaluation of the developing curriculum and ongoing measurement of student achievement have also been built into this project.

This story illustrates that steady funding must be found from a reliable source to sustain a project of this magnitude, as development is a long, slow process. Such a project should involve a cross-section of experts and representatives from groups who have an interest in the fitness and health of youth, to ensure that the curriculum is both appropriate and well supported. In fact, the consortium has consciously chosen to involve large numbers of teachers and students in visible activities that publicize the program. This is done in the belief that politicians and other stakeholders need sufficient information, including evidence of schools' involvement in the project and indicators of appropriate student achievement, to enable them to be strong, long-term advocates.

MI-EPEC materials will be offered to teachers in Michigan first, but the K–5 materials may become available to other states as early as the beginning of 1998.

If you would like to have your name included on the mailing list to receive information regarding MI-EPEC, please contact either Dr. Charles Kuntzleman or Dr. Paul Vogel at the address and phone number listed at the beginning of the story.

The PATH Program

Dr. Paul Fardy
Professor and Director of PATH
Ann Azzollini, Denise Agin, and
 Shayne Kohn
Graduate Assistants
Queens College
Department of Family, Nutrition,
 and Exercise Science
65-30 Kissena Boulevard
Flushing, NY 11367-1597
718-997-2714

▪ Physical Education
▪ Personnel Training
▪ Evaluation

Program Objectives

- To promote better health behaviors, increase health knowledge, reduce risk factors for cardiovascular disease, and improve cardiovascular fitness in adolescents
- To evaluate the effects of the program on adolescents, and to find differences between genders and ethnic groups that might affect program delivery

Program at a Glance

PATH (Physical Activity and Teenage Health) was created to help adolescents improve their cardiovascular fitness, health knowledge, and health-related lifestyles. Components of the program include participation in physical activity as well as the teaching of fitness, nutrition, and health concepts. The program has been pilot tested and is now being used in five New York high schools, one in urban Queens County, one in suburban Westchester County, and three in the rural upstate New York county of Schoharie.

Program Background

The PATH program is presently reaching 4,500 high school students in nine different schools, both within and outside New York City. The ethnic mix in the city schools is approximately 30 percent African American, 30 percent Hispanic, 30 percent Asian, and 10 percent white. Most students are from lower middle-class families. Demographic specifics for the rural settings were not available.

Beginnings of the PATH Program

The PATH program was initiated by Dr. Paul Fardy, a professor at Queens College with an interest in primary prevention of cardiovascular disease for minority populations. From looking at the literature in the field, it was clear to Paul that the least amount of prevention work had been done at the high school level, a critically important period for the establishment of healthy lifestyles.

The main purposes of the PATH program are to promote better health behaviors, increase health knowledge, and improve cardiovascular fitness in teens. The program began with screenings of minority high school students at a single high school. Screening results were shown to school officials and used to develop a pilot intervention. After reaching an agreement that the program could be run as a randomly assigned intervention so results could be used for research, he expanded the program to other schools.

Paul has been able to support and expand the program through collaboration with a number of agencies. He first had to apply to the New York City Board of Education for permission to run the program. Since that time he has kept the board apprised of the program's progress and has, in turn, received contributions (either monetary or in-kind) that support the program. The continuing relationship has also allowed Paul to be involved in advising the board on related issues. The New York State Health Department has provided additional funding to expand the program from one to three schools and then to five. Finally, exercise equipment was donated to the program by Operation FitKids, a private foundation (see Success Story 6 for more on Operation FitKids).

Program Content

Each 25-minute PATH class consists of 20 minutes of physical activity followed by 5 minutes of discussion of health and fitness information. The original PATH program focused on circuit training, which included strength training and aerobic activities using exercise machines, but it now includes a choice among several types of aerobic activity, such as step training, running, and walking, to accommodate schools that don't have exercise equipment. The core of the five-minute discussion is a lesson from the student workbook that covers basics of heart health, cardiovascular fitness, nutrition, stress, and the effects of smoking on the heart. It also contains some of the questionnaires used for pre- and posttesting. A teacher's manual is provided to instructors.

Classes meet three to five times a week for about 14 weeks, and pre- and posttesting is done with the students. PATH lessons can be incorporated into existing physical education classes or used on their own.

Program Support

To start the program at each school, Paul and his staff set up in-service trainings with the physical education teachers. For continuing support, trained college students from Queens College assist the teachers on a regular schedule. In some schools, this function is served by high school students from leaders' clubs, who are trained by the physical education teachers.

Once the program is under way, each school is responsible for its own program. However, one of Paul's two graduate assistants visits on a regular basis to observe and help teachers with the program, and teachers may call Paul directly to discuss their concerns.

Program Research and Results

From the beginning Paul has been collecting data on program participants in a number of areas, including the following:

- Height and weight
- Body mass index
- Percent body fat
- Blood pressure
- Serum cholesterol
- Cardiovascular fitness measured by estimated maximal oxygen uptake from step test recovery heart rates
- Questionnaire on demographics, lifestyle, family health history
- Multiple-choice test of healthy heart knowledge
- Stress questionnaire for adolescents

With this information he tracks the effects of the program and looks for differences between genders and ethnic groups that might help him adjust the program design to make it more effective. One controlled trial found that participation in the program was associated with significant improvement in health knowledge test scores for all students and, for girls, significant improvements in dietary habits, cholesterol levels, and cardiovascular fitness.[1]

PATH has received a commendation from the President's Council on Physical Fitness and Sports and won a competitive award from the New York State Health Department. The American College of Sports Medicine (ACSM) named it as the most outstanding program in the country in meeting the federal government's *Healthy People 2000* objectives.

Students are enthusiastic about PATH, and attendance has grown through word of mouth. Paul says he is amazed by how even students who score poorly on their pretests are interested in knowing if they've improved by the end of the program. He feels that the PATH program has opened many students' eyes to something new: how to take better care of themselves.

Improvements continue to be made in the program. The student workbook used in the program is updated every year. This year the students will be formally surveyed to find out what they think about the program. Paul hopes that the program can next be expanded to cover all the schools in Queens.

Conclusion

The PATH program has helped adolescents become more physically active, and provide them with information on fitness and nutrition. Paul attributes

---

[1] Fardy, P.S., R. White, K. Haltiwanger-Schmitz et al. 1996. Coronary disease risk factor reduction and behavior modification in minority adolescents: The PATH program. *Journal of Adolescent Health*, 18: 247-253.

much of the program's success to two factors. First, using college students or peers as helpers provides good role models for those enrolled in the program. Students who might have trouble relating to adults can be reached through these helpers. Second, much time was spent gradually developing this program. After the initial planning in 1988, the program went through two pilot screenings and a pilot project before it reached its present state.

Another strength of the program is that teachers were given plenty of help with materials, training, and ongoing staff support. A key to the program's growth has been Paul's close collaboration with groups such as the New York City Board of Education, the New York State Health Department, and Operation Fit Kids.

If you are interested in seeing a sample of the participant manual used in the program, contact Dr. Paul Fardy at the address or phone number shown at the beginning of this story.

For more detailed information on the PATH program and its results, read the following articles or chapters:

Fardy, P.S., R. White, L. Clark et al. 1994. Coronary risk factors and health behaviors in a diverse ethnic and cultural population of adolescents: A gender comparison. *Journal of Cardiopulmonary Rehabilitation*, 14: 52-60.

Fardy, P.S., R. White, L. Clark et al. 1995. Health promotion in minority adolescents: A Healthy People 2000 pilot study. *Journal of Cardiopulmonary Rehabilitation*, 15: 65-72.

Bloomsburg Area
School District Program

10

Bloomsburg, Pennsylvania

Suzann Schiemer
Physical Education Department Head and
K–5 Physical Education Specialist
Bloomsburg Area School District
728 East Fifth Street
Bloomsburg, PA 17815
717-784-5000

■ Physical Education

Program Objectives

- To provide a comprehensive, student-centered physical education program that meets the developmental needs of all students
- To use assessment and technology as a means to achieve program goals and objectives

Program at a Glance

The physical education program of the Memorial and Beaver Main Elementary Schools provides student-centered learning based on the results of assessment done every class session. With a foundation of a cutting-edge curriculum and the use of innovative activities and technology, instructors get the most out of limited class time. Extracurricular physical activity opportunities supplement the physical education program.

Program Background

The Bloomsburg Area School District centers around Bloomsburg, Pennsylvania, a rural town of about 12,500 that is also the site of Bloomsburg University. It is a lower middle-class area whose residents have a strong sense of community. Memorial Elementary School has between 550 and 600 students and is located in town, which means that more out-of-school activities are available through the university, the local Y, and other youth-oriented groups. Beaver Main Elementary has 130 students and is located outside of town. While those students have less access to in-town activities, they do have opportunities to participate in 4-H Clubs.

Curriculum Development

In the early 1980s, Sue Schiemer felt that it was time to improve her school's elementary physical education program. Sue set out to create a performance-based curriculum guide that incorporated cutting-edge ideas on teaching physical education. The aim of the program was to teach motor skill development for games, sports, aquatics, and dance, as well as knowledge and performance of exercise, fitness measurement, and personal fitness program design. The curriculum covered the psychomotor, cognitive, and affective domains with assessments for each area:

- Psychomotor skills were to be observed for isolated critical elements of each skill, combinations of critical elements, and use of the skills in authentic situations such as game play.
- Cognitive skills were to be measured with written questions before and after each unit, written quizzes, homework, and oral question-and-answer sessions.
- Affective elements were to be assessed with student self-evaluations, peer evaluations, and teacher observations.

A portfolio with materials from every year's physical education class was also to be created for each student. It would include written assessments of knowledge of concepts, sample class or homework assignments, skills checklists, the student's appraisal of the physical education program at the beginning and end of each year, and any special recognition awards.

The final curriculum guide included target outcomes for the lessons, units, and overall program, along with suggested activities and sample assessment methods with criteria for skill mastery. Although specific activities were included, each teacher is free to use whatever activities and teaching methods he or she likes, as long as the lesson outcomes are covered.

A Typical Lesson

The instructor tells students what the main activities for the day will be as they come in the door. They then break into learning teams, go to equipment that's color-coded for their team, and begin practicing a previously learned skill.

Once all the children have arrived, the teacher has each learning team lead warm-up activities. These are performed through three stations: one for aerobic fitness, one for flexibility, and one for strength. At the fourth station, each child performs the previous lesson's skill. The teacher assesses how well the children performed the skill, then checks that the activities selected for developing aerobic fitness, flexibility, or strength meet the needs of the students.

If the assessment shows that the children need to analyze the movement more or see it performed well, the instructor may choose to use an electronic visual aid. For instance, if the skill being learned is punting a ball, one class might see a video on proficient punting form. Another one might see a computer graphics demonstration of the critical elements of a proficient kick. These aids, which catch students' interest, take only 5 to 10 minutes of class.

The students then practice whatever critical element of a skill is necessary for improvement, either one not yet mastered or a new one presented by the instructor. Usually the practice is presented as some type of game. For example, if the aim is to practice punting distance, the game might be to punt a ball to hit the wall from one of various distances marked on the floor. The student chooses which distances to attempt and, if the child succeeds, he or she scores a point. However, even though there is one game, students can choose to play it in different ways. A pair of partners or small groups can decide if they want to compete against each other, cooperate with each other to reach a certain point score, or individually try for personal best scores. Each child also can decide what size and shape of ball he or she wants to use. Some may prefer the success they can get kicking a lighter ball; others may want the challenge of using a heavier one.

During practice the teacher observes and helps individual children. Students often are given the option of pairing up during practice to assess and help each other. Each one analyzes the other's movement, scoring it on paper and assisting the partner in improving technique.

At the end of practice each child is given a short pencil-and-paper assessment on the critical elements of the skill practiced. The assessment might cover the three critical elements of a particular movement are, or how to properly perform a certain element. When the instructor sees the children trying to mimic the correct skill element in order to answer the question, it's obvious that the children are learning how to analyze movement.

At the end of each class, the teacher records on a skills checklist three scores for each child's performance during that session: one for motor skill, one for concepts learned, and one for attitude and cooperative social interactions. Additional comments might also be included.

At a later time the teacher inputs the data onto a computer through software that allows educators to handle classroom management, student achievement, and performance projection. Data inputting can be made even simpler with the use of a message pad computer. The teacher can record each student's performance on critical elements of a skill; note how many observations were made during class; keep track of scores for motor skill, concepts, and attitude; and record attendance data. This information can later be sorted into reports such as daily summaries, lists of observations of particular aspects of performance, and lists showing students who have mastered each aspect of performance. This helps the instructor design appropriate follow-up lessons, identify students who need extra help or additional activities, and track student progress.

Extracurricular Activities

Because students don't get P.E. every day, Sue has tried to supplement it with additional outside activities:

- Manipulative equipment is made available for all students at recess.
- A Jump Rope for Heart event is held each year to benefit the American Heart Association.
- A rope-skipping team called the Pouncing Panthers is open to all children. The team meets once a week to learn skills and be active. Children are placed in different practice sessions depending on their needs and learning styles.
- The Pennsylvania Governor's Challenge Fitness/Education Award Program is offered; an award is given to students who participate in 48 hours of physical activity, hold a B average, and take part in a community service activity.
- The Fit n' Fun program gives families the opportunity to purchase fitness and athletic equipment at lower prices, with the school getting a certain amount of free equipment depending on the size of the families' total order.

Conclusion

This physical activity program is well thought-out and organized, uses technology, and assesses progress and skill mastery at each session. Yet its purpose isn't to show how efficient a system can be; ultimately, its purpose is to make physical education both more effective and more enjoyable.

Some of the questions that the children are asked during assessment point this out. For instance, the assessment before beginning a unit asks children not only questions such as "How well do you think you do this activity?" but also "Do you like doing this activity?" and "Is there anything you don't like about this activity?" In the end-of-the-year assessment, students are asked what they liked about this year's classes, what was different from last year, and how they felt about class.

The Bloomsburg physical education program is a good model for designing a program that is both student-centered and effective. It shows how a small school district can achieve excellence when teachers plan carefully and have a sincere desire to help children learn at their own pace.

Cabell Midland High School Program

11 — Ona, West Virginia

Bane McCracken
Department Chair, Physical Education
  Department
Cabell Midland High School
2300 U.S. Route 60, East
Ona, WV 25545
304-743-7415

■ Physical Education
■ Health Education
■ Parental Involvement

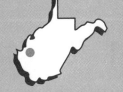

Program Objectives

- To help students develop the skills needed to successfully participate in various outdoor recreation activities
- To offer health and fitness program that students and parents can attend together
- To expose all students and interested members of the community to many aspects of fitness

Program at a Glance

The Cabell Midland High physical education department offers students a unique outdoor recreation class that combines learning physical skills for lifetime leisure activities with practical math, reading, and writing skills. It also focuses on wellness for students and the community through a Family Fun Fitness Night and an annual Fitness/Wellness Fair.

Program Background

Cabell Midland High School is in the rural village of Ona, West Virginia. Students come from a mix of backgrounds; many of their parents work in heavy or light industry, some are farmers or work in logging, and some have white-collar jobs and commute to larger cities. The student population is 2,083.

Outdoor Recreation Course

This course was developed four years ago because Bane McCracken, Cabell Midland's physical education department chair, saw that what physically active people do for recreation isn't addressed by the traditional physical education program. He wanted students to become aware of the many wonderful recreation opportunities available in West Virginia and skilled enough to take advantage of them. And he wanted noncompetitive students to have opportunities to become active outside of competitive sports.

So Bane developed a semester-long course that introduces students to six different forms of outdoor activities: downhill skiing, mountain biking, hiking, fly fishing, wilderness survival/orienteering, and whitewater rafting.

Because Cabell Midland High School uses block scheduling, this course meets five days a week for 90 minutes a day. This allows for at least 30 minutes of physical activity (such as hiking, biking, or performing individual conditioning programs) each day and still leaves plenty of time for other instructional activities.

Topics covered include the elements of fitness and how to stay fit. Students are asked to imitate performing various skills, think about what types of fitness would be necessary to perform them, then assess their own personal levels of fitness and create their own exercise prescription. As part of this process, students' body composition is measured and the students take part in the President's Challenge Physical Fitness Test.

This course doesn't just focus on physical skills; instead, Bane has students create portfolios that include reading, writing, and math assignments related to real-life outdoor activity situations. For example, the students may read an article on hiking, discuss it, and write their reflections about it. They might measure out how long their stride is, then calculate how many steps it would take to go a certain distance. Another time they may look at maps of various areas in West Virginia to locate trails they might want to hike, or even mark their own trails on blank maps.

One way Bane keeps students interested is by using electronic technology. He uses commercial videos to introduce activities and demonstrate techniques. He often videotapes students as they practice physical skills and then has them self-assess their performances, according to criteria they've been given. Students use the Internet for some lessons. For instance, one assignment for downhill skiing is finding and recording information from the home pages of states where skiing is popular.

Class activities require students' active thinking and involvement. During the downhill skiing unit students take a pretend budget of $500, go through a ski clothing and equipment catalog, and decide how that "money" should be spent. For fly tying, each student is required to choose and actually tie a fly. During the mountain biking segment, students repair bikes once a week. Finally, students can opt to take part in a ski trip and rafting trip during the semester.

Class size for this course is limited to no more than 30 students. Bane keeps all of them busy by dividing the class into four teams. At any given time one or two of the teams may be involved in physical activity while the others are involved in instructional activities. This reduces the amount of equipment or materials that need to be available at any one time.

Bane has supplied some of the necessary materials, such as the bike repair tools, on his own, and purchased others, such as fly-tying kits. He was especially lucky to be able to get a deal on 30 mountain bikes. He used to be a bike racer, and a fellow racer who owned a local bike shop was able to get in touch with Diamondback and get a price break on them.

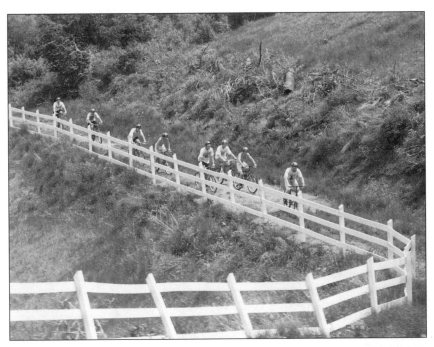

The outdoor recreation course, which includes downhill skiing, mountain biking, hiking, fly fishing, orienteering, and whitewater rafting, is a physical education program that helps students learn, be physically active, and have fun.

The nature of the activities taught in this class has raised some concerns about liability. Bane has consulted with a lawyer and developed guidelines about this. As with any program that involves physical activity and thus the potential for accidents, it is important that safety guidelines be established and followed to provide a safe experience for the participants. Steps such as establishing skill progressions to make sure students are well prepared, matching skill level, experience, and physical abilities to the appropriate activities, and searching the facilities or areas being used for potential hazards are just a few examples. Teachers should check with their school district's attorneys to help establish appropriate guidelines for their programs. While extra caution is warranted, the course is well worth it as it gives students the opportunity to try activities and develop enough skills to do them on their own.

As far as using the portfolio method for grading students, Bane says that he has been doing it for four years now and has not found it to be too difficult. He sits down with each student periodically during the course and reviews his or her portfolio materials. If something isn't done well, Bane asks the student to redo it. By the time the end of the semester comes, Bane has a good sense of how each student has performed. He says it takes him no more than a few minutes to review each portfolio at the end of the semester to determine a grade.

Family, Fun, Fitness Night

This is a new, six-week program developed by Drexena that meets one evening a week for 90 minutes. It's open to students, their parents, and the community at large. Each meeting includes a guest speaker, exercise activity, and group activity. For example, after a guest speaker talked about physical activity programs, the group as a whole went to the gym and were taught how to check their heart rate. This was followed by several fitness activities, such as working out at the Wellness Center or doing step aerobics.

At the beginning of the program, an instructor using high school student volunteers as models demonstrates proper use of the exercise machines in the Wellness Center. At each subsequent meeting an instructor is always available to help newcomers and to make sure participants are using the equipment safely and correctly.

All the guest speakers are volunteers from community agencies such as the local hospital, YMCA, and health center. School facilities, which include two gyms, an auditorium, and a fitness center, are used for activities. The program is run at very little cost and takes only about a week's worth of work to organize.

Students have been encouraged to bring their parents to the program so they could be supported at home in meeting their health and fitness goals. However, so far students have come mainly by themselves, and adult participants have come from the community at large. Participation has been good to this point; 60 people came to the second session.

This is a program that is evolving to meet the needs of the community. For instance, in the beginning there were no plans to include any strength training in the program. However, one of the participants asked an instructor about exercises for the upper body, they started doing the exercises with light weights from the Wellness Center, and soon many other people joined in. It's now become a regular part of the program.

Fitness/Wellness Fair

A Fitness/Wellness Fair is held each year to give students access to health and fitness information, as well as to expose them to new or special activities not covered in the present curriculum. It also is open to invited groups in the community, such as seniors and various organized clubs.

Some of the fair activities include:

- Body composition measurement (by several methods)
- Diet analysis
- Healthy snacks
- American Cancer Society and American Red Cross information displays
- Spirometer measurement of lung capacity
- Strength and fitness analysis
- Fitness demonstration of steps and slides
- Displays from a bike shop, hiking outfitter, sporting goods store, and canoe and kayak store
- Information from the local hospital and the mental health center
- Fly tying, clogging, and jump rope exhibitions

All of the activities are presented by community members representing national and local agencies, nearby Marshall University, fitness-related retail stores, and the local hospital. Because of these in-kind contributions, few costs are involved. Set-up is done by physical education students, and organizing tasks are split between the physical education and health education departments.

About 800 students and about 50 visitors from the community usually visit the fair. Bane is disappointed that the local media haven't given the fair much publicity, but he continues to try. He also attempts to get new activities for the fair each year such as fly tying, which was extremely popular last year.

Conclusion

The Cabell Midland outdoor recreation course is a good example of how a physical education class can both meet students' present needs for physical activity and prepare them for the future. In this class, students are provided ample time to be active daily through enjoyable activities. They also are given realistic active learning assignments that help them gain the knowledge and skill necessary to participate in several types of lifelong physical activities.

The other two programs described—Family, Fun, Fitness Night and the Fitness/Wellness Fair—are low-cost methods to get more parent support for students' physical activity and to offer students personal health information and an opportunity to learn about new forms of physical activity.

Mitchell High School Adventure Education Program

12

Colorado Springs, Colorado

Jill Sims
Physical Education Teacher and
   Health Teacher
Mitchell High School
1205 Potter Drive
Colorado Springs, CO 80909
719-520-2750
   Environment
   Physical Education

Program Objectives

- To offer students the opportunity to learn the skills necessary for life-long leisure pursuits
- To engage students in physical activities that will develop their trust in others, confidence, cooperation, and teamwork

Program at a Glance

Inspired by reading about and seeing the positive changes in teens involved in adventure activities, Jill Sims decided that adventure courses should become part of the physical education curriculum at Mitchell High. She is working to develop a variety of classes and is successfully obtaining grants to help defray the start-up costs of equipment. Money for a climbing wall came as a result of a grant proposal developed jointly by students and teachers.

Mitchell High School has a student population of 1,263, about a quarter of which consists of minorities. The school is in an urban area, and most students come from a lower- to middle-class background.

The Adventure Education Program

Jill Sims, one of the physical education teachers at Mitchell High School, first got the idea of starting an adventure education program from her experiences working with campers in the summer. An avid camper and outdoorsperson, Jill could see firsthand how campers learned responsibility, trust, and cooperation through their outdoor group activities. She became interested enough to take a course in challenge activities for coaches in the summer of 1996. That September she started working on developing an adventure activities curriculum for her high school.

Jill wants to provide a variety of programs that appeal to all students. She started in 1997 with in-line skating (leading to in-line basketball and roller hockey) and scuba diving. Next will be a climbing course conducted indoors on a climbing wall. She also is preparing an outdoors course that would combine canoeing, orienteering, camping, and fishing, and her future plans include a ropes course and mountain biking.

For now, each course is offered for nine weeks, meeting every day for 50 minutes. In the future Jill may create a semester-long class that offers an introduction to each of these activities. Students will also be able to sign up for more than one class. Another option will be for students to join an after-school program to be supervised by Jill and other certified staff.

In each course students will first have a chance to practice their skills at school, then have opportunities to get outside and try them in a real-life setting. All of these activities will be done in a group. The purpose is not just to teach students leisure activities they can pursue all their lives, but also to put them into situations in which they need to problem-solve as a group.

Jill is aware that liability can be a problem with these activities, so she has worked with her school district's risk management program to develop safety guidelines. Each student must sign a waiver before taking part in an adventure activity.

Jill had been coaching at Mitchell High, but she has given up those duties in order to concentrate on the adventure courses. Next year, when the program starts up, teaching those courses will be a large part of her physical education teaching load.

Finding the Resources

One of the problems with starting an adventure curriculum is that the equipment needed is costly. Jill applied for a number of grants to meet this need.

The first and key grant was a request for money to buy a climbing wall. Grant money was being offered by the Colorado Department of Education. Jill sought student input by posting a sign asking for help in developing the grant. Three students from the student council volunteered, and they met with Jill and another teacher, Norma Neessen, a number of times. Each student researched and then wrote a section of the grant, and they all reviewed each other's work. The grant, one of 114 proposals submitted from all over the state, was one of 34 that were finally approved for funding.

Jill is now using the work done on this grant to create grant proposals for other parts of the adventure program. She recently obtained a grant from a joint project by the National Association for Sport and Physical Education and Roller Blade called "Skate in School." Hers was one of 250 proposals funded. As a result the school will receive 40 pairs of roller blades and all the accompanying protective gear, plus lesson plans.

Jill is continuing to pursue at least five other grants. She says that, once you have the basic information for an initial grant and get a list of all the grants available, you can try a lot of possible funding sources.

Besides grants, Jill has obtained valuable in-kind contributions. A local outdoor outfitters store, Grand West Outfitters, has donated an overhang for the climbing wall and will be donating time to train instructors on climbing technique. In return the school will allow the store to offer people in the community a climbing course and use the school's climbing wall. Another local store, Diver's Reef, is giving the school a break on what they normally charge for providing on-site instruction in scuba diving.

For the outdoor portion of the adventure course, Jill has arranged a swap between the school and the Boy Scouts of America. In return for allowing scouts to use the school's climbing and in-line skating equipment, the Scouts will allow students to use Scout camping and canoeing equipment, as well as the rifle and archery range, at their nearby camp on Lake George. In addition, the Colorado State Division of Wildlife will be providing curriculum and instruction on fishing and some fishing poles for casting and fly fishing, and stocking a lake for a fishing event (or a day of fishing).

Finally, the school district itself has contributed $1,500 for Jill to use as she wishes to support the programs. The district maintenance fund also will pay for equipment maintenance.

Course Structure

The proposed climbing class provides an example of how the adventure classes will be run. Each class will be broken down into two or three small groups of eight to twelve students, forming teams. Students who are climbing will be supported and encouraged by the others on their team. Some team members will be responsible for belaying, or holding the rope that supports the climber. Others may help guide the climber by pointing out footholds or handholds that aren't visible to him or her.

Each student will be responsible for keeping a journal. Students will use it to describe what they did during each class, how they felt about what they did, and how well they are achieving the goals they've set for themselves.

Instructors will check each student's climbing skills at the beginning and end of the course. He or she also will keep notes on the student's attitude and behavior in class, since citizenship scores are given at Mitchell High School as well as achievement grades.

After the course the students will have a chance to evaluate it. Parents will receive questionnaires to identify how the course may have changed their children's attitudes and behavior at home, and teachers will fill out questionnaires on students' attitudes and behavior in the classroom.

Part of the grant proposal for the climbing wall funding included plans to track one out of every five students at 6, 12, and 18 months after the class on their academic and physical fitness progress. The hope is to find reductions in discipline problems, better grades, and better citizenship scores for students who have participated in adventure activities.

Sharing With the Community

Jill hopes that the climbing wall and some of the other activities may be made available to interested people in the community as well as students. Grand West Outfitters plans to offer a climbing course to develop interest in climbing as an activity. A climbing course will be developed for the adult education program at another community school.

Conclusion

The Mitchell High adventure education curriculum is an example of a physical education course that teaches students activities they can pursue out in the community. Through active learning, students develop the necessary skills and confidence to participate in many types of enjoyable physical activities. This program also gives students and community members the chance to try several outdoor activities outside of school hours.

Although the start-up costs are high, Jill has found ways to fund the adventure education program by actively pursuing grants and forming mutually beneficial partnerships with local adventure activity-related businesses, organizations, and agencies.

If you are interested in more information on grant lists or want to see a sample grant proposal or a course description, contact Jill Sims at the address or phone number shown at the beginning of this story.

Madison Junior High School Program

13   Naperville, Illinois

Phil Lawler
District Coordinator
1000 River Oak
Naperville, IL 60565-2700
630-420-6408

■ Environment
■ Physical Education
■ Parental Involvement
■ Personnel Training

Program Objectives

- To change the physical education program to emphasize cardiovascular fitness rather than sports
- To challenge each student at his or her ability level
- To help students make lifestyle changes to enhance their health, using technology to provide feedback
- To involve parents in promoting physical activity for their children

Program at a Glance

The physical education staff at Madison Junior High took a traditional sports-oriented physical education program and transformed it into one focusing on health-related fitness. The staff uses innovative methods to motivate and involve students and their parents in physical education. Teacher training and collaboration with the community also helped strengthen the program.

Program Background

Madison Junior High is located in Naperville, a far western suburb of Chicago. This rapidly growing community of over 100,000 is upper middle class. Enrollment at Madison Junior High during the 1995–96 school year was 915 students.

Program Description

The five members of Madison Junior High's physical education staff had heard a lot about how unfit American children were, that many children were obese and few could meet national fitness standards. In 1988 they resolved to do something about it at their own school. With the support of their building principal, and using *Healthy People 2000* as their guide, they decided to examine every activity in their program to see if it helped students become and stay fit. Over time they made the following changes.

FITNESS-FOCUSED AND PRACTICAL

The staff's foremost concern was that class activities promote cardiovascular fitness. Each activity was altered as needed to meet this criterion. For example, flag football had always been taught with teams of 10, using a huddle before plays. However, the large teams resulted in only a few players having the opportunity to touch the ball and the huddles cut down on the time available for actual physical activity. To counteract this, staff reduced teams to three-on-three or four-on-four and eliminated the huddle, giving all students a chance to be more active. Rules and strategies for the regular game were still taught, but the smaller teams allowed for a greater focus on throwing and catching skills and developing cardiovascular fitness.

Another discovery the staff made was that, although they knew why certain activities were being taught, the students didn't. They decided to give students the rationale behind class activities. For instance, at the beginning of the flag football unit, students were told that, even though they might not often play football, it is a good vehicle for learning throwing and catching skills that can be transferred to other sports. The teachers also talked about the fact that football is a large part of American culture. In relationships with others, whether personal or career-oriented, it could well be an advantage to understand and be able to talk about football.

PHYSICAL EDUCATION FOR EVERYONE

Another change that Madison's staff made was to shift emphasis from a traditional, competitive sports curriculum that appealed to only some stu-

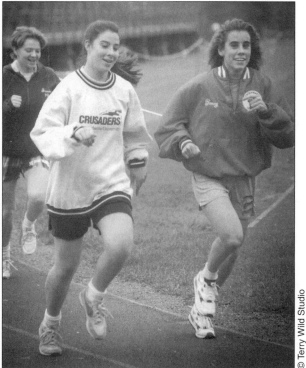

Students run for 12 minutes once a week for three weeks. Running for time rather than distance helps balance a program designed to motivate both those who are physically fit and those who are not.

dents to a balanced program that motivated and challenged all students. They wanted to challenge the fit to be better and encourage the less fit to work harder.

One activity that filled the bill, while developing cardiovascular fitness, was running. Every student does a 12-minute run once a week for three weeks. Running for time rather than distance gives faster athletes the challenge of covering more distance in the same time and saves slower ones from being embarrassed by trailing in at the end of the pack.

In the fourth week, students run a mile as a test of their improvement. Many students have found the mental barrier to running a mile almost more formidable than the physical one. Yet, with teachers' encouragement, almost all have been able to achieve it.

Other aspects of the Madison program that encourage the less fit to participate are grading on personal best efforts or based on goals rather than in comparison with other students, and using an extra credit system. The extra credit system allows students to gain points toward a higher grade by performing physical activity outside of class. This can be walking or running a mile, riding an exercise bike five miles, or using home exercise equipment.

LIFESTYLE CHANGES ASSISTED BY TECHNOLOGY

Another thrust of the Madison physical education program is to make students aware of their current health status, sometimes through the use of technology such as heart monitors and computers, and to encourage them to develop better exercise and nutrition habits.

The Madison staff conducts health-related fitness testing for all students at the beginning and end of the school year. Each student receives a computer printout that shows his or her level of fitness for each fitness component and gives a brief description of the component and how it affects daily living. Students are graded on their personal improvement and not on how their scores compare to others.

Students are encouraged to have their blood pressure and cholesterol checked, and last year a cardiologist offered on-site cholesterol testing for all students. Four hundred students took part in the screening. This partnership also benefited the cardiologist, who does research on children's cholesterol levels.

Heart rate monitors are available for students' use so they can track their heart rate as they work out. After the students exercise, instructors download the data from the monitors into a computer so a printout can be made showing students' heart rates at five-second intervals during the workout. This has not only proven to be a good incentive for students to improve their performance, but it also has shown the staff how hard the students really are working. Instructors have found that in some cases a student who doesn't appear to be exercising very hard may actually be working at a high heart rate.

Other school departments at Madison have addressed students' nutritional needs. The home economics department does a computer analysis of each student's diet, and the school cafeteria offers a low-fat lunch line.

PARENT INVOLVEMENT

One of the goals of the Madison staff is to get parents interested and involved in getting their children to be more physically active. One way they've tried to promote this is by giving students extra points for working out at home with a parent. They also have students take their fitness testing printouts home and, with their parents, set goals for each of the fitness components. Parents must certify completion of the goals.

With students who have low fitness, staff members send home student's heart rate monitor printout for parents to see their child's fitness level. They then provide those parents with counseling them on how they can help their child improve his or her fitness level.

The physical education program has also been financially supported in part by parents. The Home and School group holds a magazine sale fundraiser annually, and money from that event has gone to purchase stationary bikes, heart monitors, and a two-way radio for instructors.

Teacher Training

The Madison staff saw they needed to not only change their school's program, but also to update their knowledge about physical education. To meet this need. Madison Junior High's school district sponsors an annual workshop for physical education teachers that this year had 32 speakers and 1,000 attendees. Teachers come mainly from the Naperville area, but even some out-of-state teachers attend. At the same time, nearby Warrenville High School sponsors a Cooper Aerobic Institute workshop that teachers can attend for certification. Over 150 teachers have been certified over the last three years.

Future Program Expansion

The next big addition to the Madison program will be the addition of a fitness center. It will have exercise equipment that students can use during or after school. Some of the equipment for the center was purchased used; some was purchased at discounted prices from the Fitness Factory. Much of the funding for the center comes from proceeds from a sport drink machine that was installed near the locker rooms, replacing a soft drink machine. Staff are also working on starting up some business relationships to support and improve the center, such as possibly becoming a testing center for an equipment company.

During school time all students will get a chance to use the center for one physical education class a week. After school the center may be opened not only for students, but for their parents as well. This would be done in conjunction with a parent involvement group in the community.

Conclusion

The changes the Madison Junior High staff made in their physical education program came about gradually. It took three to four years before staff could see improvements in student fitness levels. But they have been able to continue improving the program by having a clear vision and the commitment to find innovative ways to do it. By focusing on practical, lifelong skills and fitness, finding ways to motivate students, and involving parents, they have transformed a traditional physical education program into one that's enjoyable and useful for students and their families. The 1997 annual schoolwide survey of parents' satisfaction with all school subjects showed that 93 percent of the parents who responded were very satisfied or satisfied with the Madison Junior High physical education program, and 100 percent gave the curriculum a favorable rating.

Clay Organized for Wellness (COW)

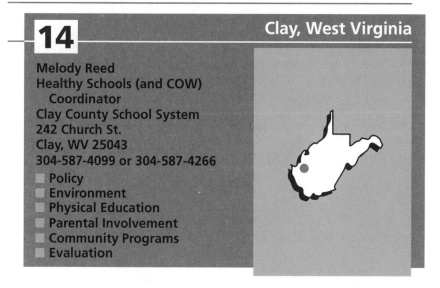

14 — Clay, West Virginia

Melody Reed
Healthy Schools (and COW)
  Coordinator
Clay County School System
242 Church St.
Clay, WV 25043
304-587-4099 or 304-587-4266

- Policy
- Environment
- Physical Education
- Parental Involvement
- Community Programs
- Evaluation

Program Objectives

- To develop community and school programs that promote healthy lifestyles and meet the needs and interests of students and other community residents
- To organize the community to identify its needs and obtain necessary resources to meet them

Program at a Glance

Through the nonprofit organization Clay Organized for Wellness (COW), Clay County has developed a comprehensive program for wellness promotion that offers a variety of physical activity services to students and community members. COW has reshaped the community's environment by creating physical activity facilities and spaces, and it has increased the amount and quality of time that students spend in physical education classes. Program decisions are made after extensive community involvement and a careful analysis of process evaluation results.

Program Background

A rural county with a population of some ten thousand, Clay is the poorest county in one of the nation's poorest states. Per capita income ranks 55th among West Virginia's 55 counties, unemployment is close to 20 percent, and there are no major industries located in the county. More than 75 percent of students are eligible for free or reduced-cost school meals, and health surveys have found high rates of obesity and other cardiovascular disease risk factors. However, Clay County has strengths that facilitate the development of a health-promotion program: a low crime rate, good schools, close families, and neighbors who watch out for one another.

Development of COW

In 1992 Clay County received a small grant from the National Association of State Boards of Education (NASBE) for planning activities to establish a comprehensive school and community health promotion program. This grant became a catalyst for Connie Harper, a registered nurse (RN) and lifelong resident of Clay County who was volunteering nursing services in the Clay schools. Along with Melody Reed, an RN who shared the same vision, Connie organized a meeting of 80 community leaders and activists. To assure good attendance, they made it a dinner meeting featuring a healthy, low-fat meal and held it at the just-completed addition to the county's middle school, a site many people were curious to see. At the meeting Melody and Connie presented the relatively dismal health statistics of West Virginia and Clay County; they were followed by guest speakers from the West Virginia Department of Education's School Health Initiative and the NASBE who discussed strategies for school-based health promotion. Each invitee was asked to complete a pledge card committing himself or herself to donating time, resources, or a health-related skill to the embryonic wellness initiative.

That 1992 meeting gave birth to a new, broad-based community coalition, Clay Organized for Wellness, that came to be known as COW. The core leadership, along with Melody and Connie, included the health department administrator, three school principals, the assistant superintendent of the school district, several health and physical education teachers, the editor of the local weekly newspaper, a town council member, a member of the parks and recreation council, a 4-H leader, and several business leaders.

COW followed a systematic problem-solving process through which community wellness needs were identified; its board members developed plans for collective solutions, established long-term goals and short-term objectives, and sought out funding sources. COW has obtained several hundred thousand dollars in grants from a variety of sources, including the state education and health agencies and the Benedum Foundation. It has taken a comprehensive approach to wellness promotion: promoting physical activity is one of its key goals, but COW activities also address other important health issues, such as nutrition, tobacco use, injury prevention, and stress reduction.

WORK SITE PROGRAM

As one of its first initiatives, COW developed workplace wellness programs for the 250 employees of the Clay school system. The school year begins, for example, with a health fair for school staff that is also open to community members. The health fair features screening for serum cholesterol, blood pressure, and obesity, as well as counseling on nutrition, physical activity, and weight control. These services have affected school staff profoundly, according to Melody Reed. "Many of them didn't realize how unhealthy they were. And then, when they made lifestyle changes, they were able to see the next year how much of an impact those changes were having on their health. It really made them buy into the program."

COW offers a variety of wellness programs at schools and other work sites in the county. In the "Six Weeks to Wellness" program, employees earn points for health-promoting actions they take, such as eating well, quitting smoking, wearing seatbelts, taking time for themselves to reduce stress, and, of course, being physically active. Participants who meet specified goals win prizes, such as athletic socks and water bottles. Participants also form three-person teams that compete to collect the most points, with winners earning cash prizes.

SCHOOL PROGRAM

Since COW turned the spotlight on the need for increasing physical activity levels of Clay County youth, Clay schools have increased the quantity and quality of time students spend in physical education classes. Each elementary school is allotted one teaching position to address the needs of high-risk youth. Local School Improvement Councils and the principals at four of the county's five elementary schools have decided to assign the teachers in this position to teach physical education, resulting in students having daily physical education. They are delighted with the results, says Melody. "Teachers report that, with the increase in physical education time, students are now paying more attention and concentrating better, there has been less absenteeism and fewer discipline problems."

Wellness centers staffed by a physician's assistant have been set up in the county's middle school and high school. School personnel have assessed and revised their health education curriculum, provided training for teachers who deliver health instruction, and established health education bulletin boards. They have involved parents through family fitness nights and incentives for family fitness activities. Elementary school classes, for example, compete to collect points for healthy actions (similar to the work site wellness program); if youngsters persuade parents or grandparents to walk or do some other physical activity with them, they get additional points. At the end of the school year, the class with the most points gets a fun field trip—one involving plenty of physical activity, of course, such as bowling, swimming, or skating.

COW helps to integrate the school and community physical activity promotion efforts. In Clay, the biggest events of the year are the Apple Festival in the fall and the Ramp Festival in the spring (a ramp is a type of wild onion). Thanks to COW, these festivals now include a 3.2-mile walk and a biking tour of about 20 miles. Students get extra credit in health and physical education courses if they participate in these activities.

The schools have also established a tobacco-free environment and worked to ensure that their food service programs comply with the standards of the Dietary Guidelines for Americans. COW is working on plans for additional after-school programs to promote physical activity, good nutrition, and a healthy lifestyle.

ENVIRONMENT

COW has created an infrastructure for physical activity in Clay County, where next to nothing previously existed. In this hilly region of winding mountain roads, it used to be difficult to even find a jogging path. Using a series of grants, COW developed the first tennis court in the county (located at an elementary school), walking paths for student and community use, two new fields for Little League programs, improvements in school playgrounds, and the community's first fitness center.

Students are building a 5,000-square-foot fitness center, funded by a federal grant for a vocational-school training program. Equipment for the center was obtained through another grant. Additional COW plans include developing another tennis court and some biking paths on low-use state roads.

COMMUNITY SERVICES

COW serves adults in the community through physical activity programs offered in school buildings after school hours. Activities include volleyball, basketball, aerobic dancing, and line dancing. Thanks to COW's efforts, Clay County has passed a clean indoor air act, and restaurants have designated nonsmoking sections and have begun promoting healthy meals. COW has also published articles on health in the local newspaper and distributed pamphlets on wellness at work sites.

Evaluation

COW has assessed the effectiveness of its programs in a number of ways. It tracks blood pressure and cholesterol levels of adult health-fair participants and the results of students' fitness tests taken in school. Reed notes remarkable improvements seen over the years on these measures.

Health-fair participants are surveyed to identify the types of physical activity programming that interest them. All participants in wellness programs are asked to identify program strengths and weaknesses. In addition, COW leaders review attendance figures to make sure they are offering community residents the types of physical activity services they desire. COW has a subcommittee on physical activity that regularly assesses the program's physical activity services.

Conclusion

Clay County's accomplishments in promoting good health were recognized in 1996 when COW won the Healthcare Forum's Healthier Communities Award in the Small, Rural, and Regional Communities category. Despite the program's successes, it still faces many challenges. Funding for various services, including Melody's position, is uncertain, and COW must continuously search for creative funding opportunities. In the meantime, COW works to make its services more self-sustaining. It obtained third-party reimbursement for some school wellness-center services, charged adults a modest fee for participating in community physical activity programs, and assessed young people a fee for participating in the county's first basketball camp. Many services are coordinated by volunteers, rather than by paid staff.

Despite the never-ending struggle to ensure that the program endures, Melody's enthusiasm has not diminished. "We've all seen so many great changes in the attitudes of community members toward health, and those attitudes are being reflected in behavioral changes," she said.

Clay County demonstrates the importance of bringing together different sectors of the community to work on overcoming barriers to physical activity. It highlights the importance of a needs assessment to rallying support, and of conducting ongoing program assessment to make sure that program services are truly meeting the needs and interests of the community. Melody advises activists in other communities that "COW can be replicated in any community where a group of citizens with common goals can come together with a vision for improving the health of the community."

University Park
Community Center

15

Portland, Oregon

Lee Jenkins
Director
University Park Community Center
9009 North Foss St.
Portland, OR 97203
503-823-3631
■ Community Programs

Program Objectives

- To offer a wide variety of physical activity services for community residents from preschoolers to senior citizens in their local community center
- To have teenagers mentor younger children in physical activity and health and, in the process, develop their own health knowledge, attitudes, and skills
- To start offering physical activity to preschoolers as forms of play and continue lifelong activity for seniors through dance and walks

Program at a Glance

The University Park Community Center offers young people an array of competitive and noncompetitive physical activities through after-school and summer programs. The Center also features an innovative program called the Health Club, which uses teenagers as physical activity and health mentors for younger children. The Center highly regards the importance of preschool activity, adult fitness, and senior physical fitness activities.

Program Background

The University Park Community Center is located in Portland's Columbia Villa / Tamarack community, the largest housing project in Oregon. The

North Portland population served is low-income and largely African American. The Center is run by Portland's Bureau of Parks and Recreation. Its staff includes a director, two program coordinators, and part-time staff as needed to help with specific activities.

Development of Center Activities

When Lee Jenkins began as director of the University Park Community Center in 1988, the place was so quiet he could hear the paint dry. Residents were too afraid of local gangs to leave their homes; in fact, just the month before Lee arrived, the Center itself was the site of Portland's first drive-by shooting. A police crackdown helped restore order to the area, and Lee set out to get the youth of the community involved in physical activity. Lee stayed after hours and showed that he really cared about the community's youth. How could he not care, he asks, being a Portland native who lived part of his childhood in Columbia Villa.

Lee knew that the quickest way to attract a crowd would be through the favorite sport of Portland's inner city youth: basketball. With the help of a few friends and associates, Lee developed a basketball team, and young people started flocking to the Center's gym. He let kids use parts of the Center that had previously been off-limits to them, including the pool tables of the Center's senior-citizen program. And, soon enough, he obtained a grant from the city's school district that enabled him to develop additional programming for the neighborhood's young people.

Center Services

University Park Community Center is now a multipurpose community center that features a preschool program, senior-citizens program, after-school program, and summer camps. Because of the low-income levels of area residents, Lee and his staff are continually working to obtain free services or grants.

The after-school and camp programs place a great emphasis on physical activity and teaching young people good sportsmanship. Physical activity services are designed to provide low-income North Portland youth with a wide variety of sports and recreational activities where they can explore their interests and discover their abilities. Activities are carefully designed to assist students in developing integrity, character, social skills, physical and mental fitness, conflict management and resolution, self-discipline, leadership, and team-building skills, as well as respect for self and others.

Activities offered in the after-school program include tumbling and gymnastics, karate, tai chi, a youth golf program sponsored by the Ladies Professional Golf Association, step aerobics, circuit training, waist busters (a workout concentrating on the stomach, hips, thighs, and back), weightlifting, basketball, soccer, flag football, and track and field. A weight room is open to older adolescents until 8:00 P.M. Summer activities include gymnastics, T-ball, bowling, dance, and a junior sports fitness camp for elementary school students.

One of Lee's favorite programs is called Urban Exposure, which gives youngsters who rarely leave the housing project a chance to take field trips to interesting places in Portland and the surrounding area. The goals of this program are to expose the children to leisure-time activities that broaden their awareness of recreational opportunities to help them make wiser choices about how to spend their spare time and money. Horseback riding, rafting, camping, fishing, racquetball, roller skating, and skiing are just a few of the different kinds of physical activities these children are exposed to through this program.

THE HEALTH CLUB

One of the most innovative programs at University Park Community Center is the Health Club, which was developed with the help of the Oregon Health Division, the Columbia Boys and Girls Club, the Health Education Program at Portland State University, and other community agencies and businesses. Like all programs offered at the Center, the Health Club is designed to facilitate skill development, self-esteem, and civic/community participation and pride.

At the heart of the Health Club are local middle and high-school students who are hired to serve as mentors for elementary school students. Their task is to organize a series of activities for the children, keeping three objectives in mind: education, physical activity, and health/nutrition. Mentors spend the first thirty minutes of every session in the library, either reading to or with their assigned children. Working on homework is also an option.

The health component deals with a variety of issues, ranging from developing social skills and positive self-image, to gaining physical and mental wellness, as well as dealing with social issues, such as drug and alcohol abuse, violence, and abstinence. Numerous assessment procedures and incentives are built into the program to keep staff, tutors, and the young children focused on program goals. For example, children are asked questions about stories they were read that day and are rewarded for their efforts in paying attention. Perfect weekly attendance is also rewarded. Lastly, at the end of each week, the Health Club participates in Urban Exposure, where the kids have an opportunity to enjoy leisure activities in an environment they might not otherwise have the chance to visit.

The Health Club offers physical activities that involve everyone, regardless of ability, age, or gender. The high-school students form positive relationships with the younger kids, which play a major role in making the kids feel safe and comfortable during any activity. The mentors not only set up activities, but are also active participants. With enthusiasm and constant encouragement, the mentors model good sportsmanship, positive attitudes, and teamwork and discourage the concept of winners and losers. Using non-competitive games, the Health Club's goal is to build self-esteem through fun and support.

Lee hires a new set of mentors each semester. He particularly looks for young people who have had problems in the past and are at high risk for having more problems in the future. Mentors are required to do a lot of personal reflection during their service and to keep a personal journal where they write about their experiences, their problems in doing their job, and the lessons they have learned. Although the Health Club is primarily designed to serve the needs of elementary school students, Lee suspects that the mentors may actually be the ones who benefit most.

Conclusion

The University Park Community Center shows that excellent programs for promoting physical activity can be implemented despite limited resources and a challenging community environment. It demonstrates the importance of offering children a wide variety of physical activity options to choose from and the value of cross-age and lifelong learning experiences.

Children's Hospital of Illinois

16

Peoria, Illinois

Suzi Lintz Boos
Manager of Youth Programs
Children's Hospital of Illinois
at OSF Saint Francis Medical Center
2265 W. Altorfer Drive
Peoria, IL 61615
309-589-5802

- Physical Education
- Health Education
- Parental Involvement
- Personnel Training

Program Objectives

- To increase physical activity through a variety of youth programs developed and sponsored by a hospital

Program at a Glance

The programs presented here illustrate how a hospital can provide community leadership in improving physical activity opportunities for children. The three programs described were all developed and sponsored by the Youth Programs department of Children's Hospital of Illinois.

Children's Hospital of Illinois at OSF Saint Francis Medical Center is a part of the health care system owned by The Sisters of the Third Order of St. Francis. The hospital is located in Peoria, Illlinois, and it serves the city of Peoria, which has a population of over 114,000 and a referral base of 750,000 spread over 22 counties. In the Peoria public school system, 55 percent of students come from low-income families.

Parent/Child Motor Skills Development Class

In 1987 Suzi Boos, a staff member of the Children's Hospital sports medicine department, designed a program to help parents help their children develop their basic motor skills. The program, which consists of 8 one-hour sessions for parents and their 18 month to 5 year old children, continues today under the name Healthy Steps.

Healthy Steps is open to anyone in the community for a fee of $45, although scholarships are available. Its goals are to help children learn efficient and effective patterns of basic motor skills and to teach parents how to facilitate their children's learning in this area. The seven motor skills taught are catching, throwing, striking, kicking, jumping, stability, and spatial awareness.

During the first session, parents watch a videotape of a Healthy Steps class in action and are taught how to evaluate and improve their child's motor skills levels. Every parent also gets the opportunity to perform each step of each motor skill. The seven subsequent sessions are devoted to parent/child activities at about 18 different movement centers. Each week the equipment layout is different. Two physical education specialists facilitate the activities.

One of the initial problems with starting the program was that people thought of hospital-based programs as being for children with illnesses or injuries. It took much promotion in local schools and preschools and to parents' organizations—even in the hospital's own birthing center—to convince people that the classes were meant for *all* young children. Once parents had experienced the classes, though, word of mouth helped get the idea across. Over the first two years about 1,200 children and adults participated in the program.

By 1996 and 1997, enrollment had risen to over 2,000. Further program expansion has been limited by space and time constraints.

Early Childhood Education Center

Because of her experience in early childhood programming, Suzi was asked to join the curriculum planning committee for the Valeska Hinton Early Childhood Education Center. This Center was designed as a model program that could spread new teaching methods to other Peoria school, day care, and Head Start programs.

Physical activity was not given priority in the new preschool's curriculum, but Suzi stayed in touch with the school and about a year after it opened, school personnel contacted her. They wanted her help in developing an effective movement training program. The school could not afford a physical education teacher and wanted a program that was integrated into the curriculum. Thus, the goal was to teach all instructors why movement education was needed and how to implement an appropriate movement education program for their children.

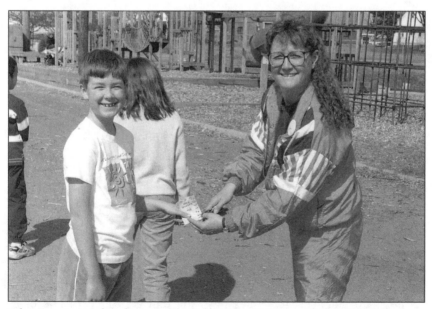

Schools reported that the use of the Feelin' Good Mileage Club built self-esteem in the children, helped them become more fit, and reduced playground arguments.

With grant funding from a local community foundation, Suzi and the school's professional development coordinator, Judy Harris Helm, developed a staff training program that public schools in the Peoria area could replicate. A large room was set aside in the preschool for movement education. Suzi and Mary Jo Jones, a fellow physical educator at Children's Hospital, held five interactive half-day workshops to teach instructors how to plan and present appropriate movement activities.

The teachers were given evaluation criteria for specific motor skills and taught how to observe those skills. Two or three skills were covered in each workshop. The skills were then reviewed at subsequent meetings or through handouts and videos. Teachers also were taught how to choose developmentally appropriate equipment for particular tasks, how to organize a lesson, and where to find resources. Between workshops, Suzi and Jo talked informally with teachers, met with Judy to evaluate progress, and then adjusted the workshops to fit the teacher's needs.

After attending several workshops, the teachers took turns planning the movement activities for all classes for two to three weeks at a time. The teacher in charge would draw up lesson plans and set up the equipment.

Children's Hospital supported this program by giving Suzi some release time for working on the program (although she also worked on her own time) and loaning equipment to the school so they could try it out before buying.

Evaluations of the program done for the grant showed significant positive changes in teachers' attitudes toward movement activities and their skills at planning lessons for physical skill development and movement activities. Since then the program has been used as a model for program planning, for teacher training, and for an Illinois program to train Special Supplemental Nutrition Program for Women, Infants, and Children (WIC) staff to conduct classes on basic motor skill development for WIC parents and their three- to five-year-old children.

Mileage Club

In 1994 Suzi started the Feelin' Good Mileage Club for elementary school children in Peoria, with start-up support from a Children's Miracle Network grant. In this program, originally developed in Michigan, children walk or run at noon, during recess, or before school, and record their mileage on a card. For every five miles they walk, they get a small plastic token to decorate their shoelaces; higher levels of mileage win them certificates and brightly colored shoelaces. Many schools add their own incentives.

Suzi had great success in recruiting schools for the Mileage Club because many school administrators knew her from earlier teacher trainings she had done; she offered to train coordinators from each school; and the Children's Miracle Network grant enabled her to offer all the program materials—posters, mileage cards, incentive items—at no cost. Her only requirements were that school administrators write a statement about why the program would work in their schools and that they assign someone to coordinate the program.

The program started in 16 schools in the fall of 1995, and, by the spring of 1996, more than 5,000 children at 26 schools were participating. Programs are coordinated by a variety of people: physical education teachers, principals, volunteer parents, and lunchroom or playground personnel. Children, parents, and teachers have written to Suzi to express how the program has improved their lives and health.

Conclusion

Children's Hospital demonstrates how a community-based institution can positively affect the health and fitness of its community. This story shows how hospitals can effectively collaborate with schools and child care centers to develop innovative programming to promote physical activity among young children.

Several articles have been published over the years describing the Children's Hospital projects in more detail. The Spring 1989 issue of *Illinois Journal of Health, Physical Education, Recreation and Dance* contains an article about the start of the Healthy Steps program. An article in the March 1996 issue of the same journal provides more detail on the work done at the Valeska Hinton Early Childhood Education Center.

Minnesota State High School Adapted Athletic Program

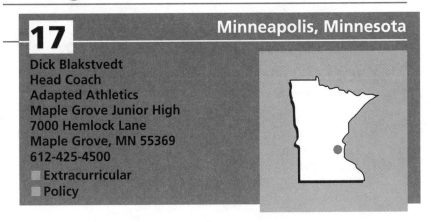

17 Minneapolis, Minnesota

Dick Blakstvedt
Head Coach
Adapted Athletics
Maple Grove Junior High
7000 Hemlock Lane
Maple Grove, MN 55369
612-425-4500
■ Extracurricular
■ Policy

Program Objectives

- To provide junior high and high school students with disabilities opportunities to participate in a school sports program

Program at a Glance

The Metro Association for Adapted Athletics is open to students who either have a physical disability, health impairment, or mental impairment that keeps them from participating in their school's sports program. Seventh through twelfth grade students participate in three sports: indoor soccer, floor hockey, and indoor softball.

Program Background

From only three teams in one sport in 1975, the Minnesota High School Adapted Athletic Program has grown to thirteen teams in three sports. It began as an independent association, but has been incorporated into the Minnesota High School League, and the program continues to grow. It brings not only physical but also psychological and social benefits to students with disabilities.

This athletic league is open to public school students with disabilities who live in the Minneapolis area. The league has two divisions, one for those with physical disabilities or health problems and one for those who are mentally impaired. Each year about 200 students with physical disabilities and 600 who are mentally impaired participate in the program.

Development of the Metro Association for Adapted Athletics

The Metro Association Adapted Athletics School Program got its start in the 1970s when Ed Prohofsky, a physical education teacher and coach, began a program that included physically disabled students at Marshall University High School in regular physical education classes. Ed developed adapted rules for play, some of which are still in use today.

In 1975 a three-team indoor hockey league for students with physical disabilities from two schools was formed in the Minneapolis area. From that beginning, the league grew to include students from 21 area schools. In the fall of 1990, a division was created for students who were mentally handicapped. The leagues were conducted by the Minnesota Association of Adapted Athletics, which was not school-supported.

The Minnesota High School League agreed to adopt the adapted league into its organization, beginning with the 1993 school year. At this point the Minnesota Association of Adapted Athletics changed its name to the Metro Association for Adapted Athletics (MAAA). A member of the High School League board now also sits on the Metro Association board, and he oversees all adapted athletic activities, including the three state tournaments held by the adapted league.

The tournaments, which are held at the same time as those for non-disabled students, have brought TV and newspaper coverage to the adapted league's tournament play. Trophies, medals, and plaques are awarded to teams and individual players as part of the tournament.

Program Structure

The MAAA program is open to students in the seventh through twelfth grades who have a disability that keeps them from participating in their school's sports program for non-disabled students. Students who are mentally impaired play in their own league. Presently three sports are offered—indoor soccer, floor hockey, and indoor softball. Combined, they run through the entire school year.

Students and their parents hear about the program from special education staff and from other students already in the program and their parents. Information about the Adapted Athletics Program is included in pamphlets on school athletics, and the schedules for team play are publicized the same as those for the non-disabled students.

Teams have an average of 14 students. Team members are expected to practice two days a week and play once a week for 8 to 10 week seasons. Practices are from $1\frac{1}{4}$ to $1\frac{1}{2}$ hours long and are structured to start with warm-ups, then move to drills for individuals, small groups, and the team. Game strategy is also discussed. Most coaches in the adapted league have a certification in adapted physical education or special education.

When asked how he learned to coach students with disabilities, Dick said, "I found out early that one of the best things I could do was to treat the students with disabilities just like any other kids. I joked with them or gave them a hard time to relieve tensions. Just like any other coach, I expect them to work hard during practice as well as in the game. I try to teach them skills that may be above their present ability level so they can strive for better things, things they may have thought were unattainable. I respect their limitations, but, more importantly, I respect them as people."

Teams travel to compete with each other, sometimes as far as 130 miles away. Game officials, who are state certified, are hired by the State High School League and are trained in adapted rules through clinics and rules meetings.

Benefits of the Adapted Athletic Program

The MAAA believes that providing opportunities for students with disabilities to play sports gives those students the chance to develop not only physically, but also socially and psychologically. Students gain self-confidence, experience leadership and teamwork, form friendships, feel part of a community, and foster self-help skills such as concentration and goal setting. They also gain the same recognition from schools for sports participation as do non-disabled athletes, such as winning athletic letters or being included at pep rallies.

Parents have also been involved and supportive in this program from the very beginning. Advocacy by parents has probably been the key factor leading to the program's growth.

Conclusion

The Minnesota State High School Adapted Athletic Program continues to flourish and grow as it meets an important need in the community. Parents' active involvement in the program has helped promote the program and obtain school support. With the adoption of the program by the Minnesota State High School League, the athletes in the adapted league have received more recognition from the community. MAAA members continue to spread the word about the adapted league by putting on exhibition games in areas that don't yet have adapted teams and sending promotional videotapes to schools.

Best of all is the boost the program gives to the athletes in the adapted program. As they learn skills, compete, and gain recognition, their self-esteem grows. They also make friends and keep them for many years. Some athletes who have graduated still come back with their old buddies to watch the present teams compete. This program has made, and will continue to make, a difference in the lives of students with disabilities.

If you are interested in obtaining a copy of the MAAA's annual conference handbook or would like a member of MAAA to talk to you about the program, contact Dick Blakstvedt at the address or phone number shown at the beginning of this story.

Stilwell Junior High
Intramural Program

18   West Des Moines, Iowa

Mike J. Macki
Intramural Program Director
Stilwell Junior High School
1601 Vine
West Des Moines, IA 50265
515-226-2770

■ Environment
■ Extracurricular Activities
■ Community Programs

Program Objectives

- To offer intramural activities to junior high and high school students who aren't on school athletic teams
- To develop students' interest in lifelong physical activity and fitness

Program at a Glance

Stilwell Junior High's intramural program is part of a collaborative effort between the school district, the Walnut Creek YMCA, and the West Des Moines Parks and Recreation Department. That collaboration supplies a wide variety of sport and fitness activities to students in Stilwell, Indian Hills Junior High, and Valley High School, providing opportunities for all those who want to participate in physical activity. These activities are offered at no cost to students and are designed to develop sportsmanship and promote a healthy lifestyle.

Program Background

Stilwell Junior High, which includes seventh and eighth grades and has a student population of 690, is part of the West Des Moines School District. Two other district schools participate with Stilwell in a cooperative intramural program: Indian Hills Junior High, with 680 students, and Valley High School, with 2,200 students. The district is in a middle-class, suburban setting, although some students also come from lower-income families.

Development of the Intramural Program

In 1994 the school board of the West Des Moines School District realized that an intramural program was needed for seventh-graders, who could not participate on school teams, and for eighth-graders who were not on regular school teams.

District administrators suggested a collaboration with the Walnut Creek YMCA and the West Des Moines Parks and Recreation Department. An intramural program was created that serviced Stilwell Junior High, Indian Hills Junior High, and Valley High School. The YMCA and the park district assist school-based intramural directors with program development; provide trained adults to serve as coaches, mentors, and officials; and handle the finances for each school's program.

This year the school board funded the program at $51,000, with $40,000 going to the YMCA and $11,000 to the Parks and Recreation Department. This money pays for the salaries of those planning and running the program, program equipment, and facilities and transportation, if needed. The money is allotted to schools according to individual program needs.

The YMCA's sports program director, Dan Weidner, generally handles the budgeting, which frees more time for program personnel to work directly with students. However, everyone involved in the intramural program wears many hats, depending on what is needed. Cooperation is at a high level, allowing the collaborators to create exciting activities that have been extremely popular with students.

Program Content

Each school's intramural activities vary slightly from each other. Activities are chosen to meet three main criteria:

- To be good alternatives to high-risk activities, such as drug use
- To develop skills and sportsmanship that can be used throughout life
- To promote a healthy lifestyle

All activities are coed. The activities offered at Stilwell during the 1997-98 school year included the following:

Fall—flag football clinic and tournament

Winter—3-on-3 basketball tournament, wrestling clinic and tournament, basketball shootout, girls' basketball clinic, volleyball clinic

Spring—softball clinic, baseball clinic, street hockey clinic and tournament, danceline clinic

All year round—Fitness Club

Students also participate in special outings. These were developed to introduce students to new physical activities that they usually wouldn't find in school programs and that could be pursued for a lifetime. Each outing begins with a clinic to teach the necessary skills over several weeks, building up to an opportunity to perform the activity in a real-world setting.

The first outing, fishing, was offered last spring. It was attended equally by both boys and girls. After the students learned and practiced the necessary skills, they got on the YMCA van and traveled to Big Creek Reservoir to do some actual fishing. The kids who participated loved the activity and this fall asked if it could be offered again.

The next outing Mike would like to offer is orienteering, but it had to be postponed when it was first scheduled because of the threat of poison ivy in the wooded setting available. Mike would like to add a new outing each year and have at least one each fall and spring. It's important, though, that planners avoid offering an activity that they can't really support. For example, they had wanted to hold a cross-country skiing outing this winter, but the snow didn't arrive at the right time and it was difficult to find an available area in which to ski.

Students are encouraged to purchase their own equipment. Instructors will tell students where they can buy equipment most economically. However, if a student can't afford it, one of the instructors will share his or her gear.

Students have attended the intramural program activities in large numbers. Adding up the number of times individuals have participated in each activity for 1996–97, Stilwell had a total of 2,506. The number for Indian Hills was 1,529, and the number at Valley High, 1,019.

One problem facing the intramural program is space availability. Sometimes there are scheduling conflicts with other school sports or programs. One way this difficulty has been resolved is by using local elementary school gyms, especially for basketball. Fortunately, the intramural program is given priority for space by the Community Education Program.

At times only six or seven students have shown up for new activities. However, those activities have not been canceled. Usually those students who participated enjoyed it enough to tell their friends, so more students showed up the next time the activity was offered .

To try to avoid this problem at Stilwell Junior High, Mike runs new activity ideas by the student council members to see if there's interest. If the program seems like a good idea, council members then support it by attending the new program and telling classmates about it.

The intramural program requires a large investment of time. Administration of the district program takes up a lot of the YMCA sports program director's full-time job. To present activities at Stilwell, Mike says it takes him about three to five hours of preparation and ten to fourteen hours of actually working with students each week. He sometimes gets to school as early as 4 or 5 A.M. to work with students in the Fitness Club or stays at school until 5:30 P.M.

Program Benefits

Students' participation in the intramural program has helped develop more than just physical skills. Many new students have made friends quickly through the intramural program. Activities such as the Fitness Club, in which each student develops his or her own fitness goals and works to achieve them, have taught students how to set and meet goals.

Mike says he's most impressed to see 35 or 40 students show up at 6:30 A.M. and work out hard in order to reach their goals. He's found that the students participating in the intramural activities don't fight or curse each other—they know what they want to do and enjoy doing it. At the beginning, no one knew how students would respond to the program, but the students have shown up and proven that this program was needed.

Future Plans

Now that the program is several years old, Mike foresees keeping the core offerings plus adding new activities such as soccer. Knowing what will be presented this year, he and his colleagues can set up a calendar of activities so students can plan ahead to attend.

Having a stable lineup of activities also will help in promoting the program. This year Mike and his colleagues set up a home page on Stilwell's website to provide information. Next year they hope to put together a brochure on the program. This would be used to inform parents and sixth-graders who are about to enter junior high about the program. It would be especially helpful for the presentation they make at the annual open house for parents at the beginning of each school year. In time they even hope to create a promotional video.

This year the program expanded to another school district and another YMCA. This has helped stimulate even more creative thinking and activity development.

Conclusion

The high level of cooperation among all the community agencies involved in this program—school, YMCA, and parks and recreation department—has allowed them to create an attractive program that draws in many students. They can offer a variety of competitive and noncompetitive physical activities to students who would not otherwise be able to participate in extracurricular school sports. This story demonstrates how a well-coordinated effort to pool community resources can result in programs that work for youth.

Family Fitness
Program

19

Arcata, California

Chris Hopper
Department Chair
Department of Health and
    Physical Education
Humboldt State University
Arcata, CA 95521-8299
707-826-3853
■ Physical Education
■ Health Education
■ Parental Involvement
■ Personnel Training
■ Evaluation

Program Objectives

- To teach children and their families about heart-healthy physical activity and nutrition
- To involve parents in helping their children become more fit

Program at a Glance

This 6- to 10-week school-based program provides children with information on physical activity and nutrition. It also invites parents to become active with their children and to change their family's diet to improve heart health.

Program Background

The first school involved in pilot testing the program, Fortuna Town School, is in a rural area. Fortuna is a working class/middle class community of 10,000 with an economy based on lumber. Many members of the community are Hispanic.

Sunset School, one of the sites of later program testing, is in Arcata, California. Its setting is also rural, and the town of 15,000 includes Native Americans.

Program Beginnings

The Family Fitness Program had its start with the desire of Bruce Fisher, 1990 California Teacher of the Year, to do a better job of teaching physical education to his fifth-graders. Bruce talked with Dr. Chris Hopper, Department Chair of Health and Physical Education at Humbolt State University, about their mutual interest in developing activities for a program that could bring about significant changes in children's fitness and health. Chris also had an interest in involving parents in improving children's fitness, and an idea was born for a program that would provide innovative physical education activities along with parent involvement.

Various program ideas were pilot tested in Bruce's school district, Fortuna Elementary School District. The program was then revised and tested at Sunset School.

Fortuna Pilot Study

The first version of the Family Fitness Program offered six weeks of heart-healthy physical education and nutrition instruction to fifth- and sixth-graders. Two classes received a home-and-school program and two were given a school-only program. Another two classes that did not participate in the program but who received the regular school physical education and nutrition instruction served as a control group.

The program was run by the classroom teachers with in-classroom assistance from Chris Hopper's graduate students. The home-and-school classes also took part in a parent involvement component with program incentives.

PHYSICAL EDUCATION

Children were given physical education instruction in school three times a week for 40 minutes each session. The content was based on the Know Your Body Program from the American Health Foundation, the Superkids-Superfit Program from the Bogalusa Heart Study, and the Physical Best Program from AAHPERD. Activities included games, gymnastics, dance, and fundamental movement. During these activities, fitness concepts were taught as appropriate. As an example, during aerobics the children learned about pulse rate and how it relates to fitness.

NUTRITION

The nutrition portion of the program was presented in two half-hour sessions at school each week. Lessons were geared toward reducing saturated fat in children's diets. Some of the topics included how to fix heart-healthy snacks and meals, how to interpret food labels, and how to make healthy food choices. Program activities for nutrition included food preparation, films, discussion, role-playing, and games. Nutrition concepts related to cardiovascular health were integrated into the lessons, and children were also taught how to discuss nutrition at home and how family nutrition could be improved.

PARENTAL INVOLVEMENT

Every week, children in the home-and-school program brought home a packet to share with their parents. The packets included exercise ideas and directions for healthy food preparation. The materials also stressed setting goals for nutrition and exercise. Points were awarded to families for activities done at home by the child with at least one parent, and the family had a weekly point goal for both exercise and nutrition. The parents filled out a scorecard every week, and the child returned it to class to have the points recorded. Small incentive items were given to children based on points earned. When the scorecard was returned, they received a sticker; if the family had reached the target point goal, they received a balloon as well. Graduate students called the parents regularly to offer support and would call if a scorecard was not returned. This support was an important part of the program and serves as a good example of how cooperation between universities and schools can work to provide experience for graduate students and help to busy teachers.

At the beginning of the program, all the family members who signed up for the program were given a T-shirt with the program logo. At the end, as part of a heart-healthy potluck dinner, each family got a certificate and a chance for a door prize. Most of the incentives were paid for by a university grant; the dinner door prizes were donated by a local sports store and fitness club.

PROGRAM RESULTS

An evaluation of the program found that, compared to a control group, children in school-only and the home-and-school programs at the end of the program scored higher on exercise knowledge and lower on the percent of calories from fat. The home-and-school children, but not the

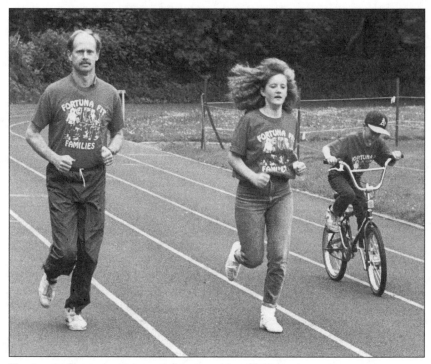

The family fitness program seems to provide schools with a way to support at home the fitness and nutrition concepts taught in school.

school-only children, scored higher than the control group on sit-and-reach flexibility and nutrition knowledge.[2]

Chris and his graduate students learned a lot about working with parents through this pilot program. First, they found that regular phone calls and the weekly scorecard were effective ways to communicate with and encourage parents. Second, they were surprised to discover that many parents felt that they had to be athletes to participate in physical activity. This program was valuable in changing some parents' attitudes. Finally, they concluded that the pilot program probably asked parents to do a little too much at home in a format that was too structured. With families' hectic schedules, parents don't have a lot of time to spend on extra activities.

---

[2] Hopper, C.A, M.B. Gruber, K.D. Munoz, and R.A. Herb. 1992. Effect of including parents in a school-based exercise and nutrition program for children. *Research Quarterly for Exercise and Sport*, 63: 315-321.

Sunset School

After implementing the program a few more times at Fortuna, Chris took a year and a half to fine-tune the school materials, making some changes in content and adjusting physical activities to ensure they kept students moving as much as possible. The revised program, which included both school and home components, was then tried at Sunset School in Arcata. The revised program was 10 weeks long, rather than 6. Two second-grade and two fourth-grade classes were involved, with one class at each level serving as the control group.

This program, unlike the earlier ones, was more of a collaboration between the university staff and the classroom teachers. The teachers were asked to deliver the program, and the university staff held seminars after school once a week for six weeks to train them on how to use the scripted lessons. Lessons were first modeled for the teachers by university staff, then the teachers practiced teaching the lessons to each other. The teachers were very positive about the training. They felt that the lessons fit in well with some of the health and physical education concepts they already were teaching, and it showed them how to run an effective physical education program.

One of the main problems with running the program was finding sufficient space and equipment. Because winters are very rainy in this area, lessons had to be created that could be done indoors in restricted space. Many innovative activities were incorporated into the revised program.

PROGRAM ACTIVITIES

The activities used in school were specifically designed to be different from traditional games. Many reinforced previously learned science concepts as well as providing physical activity. Teachers appreciated this aspect, as it made good use of limited time, and the activities encouraged children to actively participate in learning.

For example, one activity had the children jog, skip, and hop through the circulatory system of a huge heart outlined on the ground. Another had children act as blood cells transferring oxygen (represented by a ball) to other children acting as muscle cells retrieving the "oxygen" balls. The children ran to deposit the balls in a "muscle" (box) or get a new oxygen molecule (ball) from the "heart"(another box).

Nutrition activities included hands-on activities and group creative activities. In many lessons children tasted and commented on different foods.

Topics included identifying foods high in fat, salt, or carbohydrates; recognizing the importance of drinking enough water; making heart-healthy cookies; and learning how to read food labels and shop for heart-healthy foods.

At-home activities were kept simple. Suggested weekly physical activities for points were limited to aerobics, biking, walking, jogging, swimming, and jumping rope, with a few additional at-home activities for the whole family. Recipes, snacking tips, and easy-to-do food comparisons and experiments were some of the nutrition home activities.

As an added incentive to reach the goals, which were set for both physical activity and nutrition, the points families earned were considered to be "miles traveled" toward a family amusement park 500 miles away.

RESULTS OF THE STUDY AT SUNSET SCHOOL

An evaluation found that after the program the children in the treatment group scored higher than those in the control group on fitness and nutrition knowledge and number of fruit and vegetable servings consumed.[3] Children whose families had greater involvement, as measured by a higher number of points earned, were more likely to decrease their intake of cholesterol and saturated fat.

Continuation of the Family Fitness Program

Since the Sunset School study, the Family Fitness Program has been extended to six sites in Humboldt County, California. In all of these schools that have piloted the program, it has been continued in some form. Published materials for the program are now available, and Chris plans to meet with local school districts to do in-service training.

The program is fairly intensive, taking about 10 hours weekly per teacher, so Chris has suggested that it might best be used twice a year for four or five weeks. Offering it in the fall and spring would take advantage of the good weather for outside activities and keep the program from being too much of a burden for parents or teachers. Chris feels that for the program to have the greatest effect, it should be done consistently across all grades.

[3] Hopper, C.A., K.D. Munoz, M.B. Gruber et al. 1996. A school-based cardiovascular exercise and nutrition program with parent participation: An evaluation study. *Childrens Health Care,* 25: 221-235

Conclusion

The Family Fitness Program serves two purposes: It provides classroom teachers with new methods of teaching physical education and nutrition concepts, and it also offers families ways to support those concepts at home with fun nutrition ideas and physical activities they could do together.

This story demonstrates how a university-developed program can be integrated into a school system. Here, the program provided teachers with a curriculum, materials, and ample assistance to learn how to use them. As the program went through several trials, program developers learned more about what would and wouldn't work for teachers and families, and they adjusted the design until they finally came up with one that was simple enough for busy teachers and families to use successfully. Even at that, the program developers recognize that achieving success takes some intense effort on the part of teachers and parents, suggesting that programs such as these might best be used for limited time periods on a recurring basis.

If you are interested in more information on how to run the parent involvement portion of the program or want to see sample scorecards, contact Dr. Chris Hopper at the address or phone number shown at the beginning of this story.

Fairfax County Schools
FIT 4 LIFE Program*

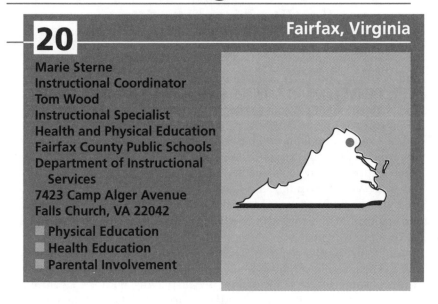

20

Fairfax, Virginia

Marie Sterne
Instructional Coordinator
Tom Wood
Instructional Specialist
Health and Physical Education
Fairfax County Public Schools
Department of Instructional
  Services
7423 Camp Alger Avenue
Falls Church, VA 22042

■ Physical Education
■ Health Education
■ Parental Involvement

Program Objectives

• To encourage students and their families to learn about and practice a healthy lifestyle

Program at a Glance

FIT 4 LIFE is a one-month wellness program offered to all students in fifth grade and above in Fairfax County public schools. Students keep track of their physical activity, nutrition, and other health habits and are awarded points depending on the type of exercise or habit and how long the physical activity was done. Performing physical activity with another family member doubles the points. At the end of the month, those who have accumulated enough points are awarded a certificate.

---

*This success story was developed from copy written by Marie Sterne.

The Fairfax County Public School District is the twelfth largest school division in the U.S. Located near Washington, DC, it serves 137,000 students in 232 schools and centers. This is largely an affluent area in which most students go on to college. The student population is 63 percent white, 14 percent Asian, 11 percent African American, and 10 percent Hispanic.

Creation of the FIT 4 LIFE Program

Fairfax County Public Schools has a Health and Physical Education Curriculum Advisory Committee consisting of elected teachers from all grade levels, parents appointed by school board members, appointed school administrators from each instructional level, and others who have special expertise in areas such as media or special education. The committee has a two-year term, and during that time they are expected to choose and complete a project that will in some way promote or improve health and physical education.

In 1994 the committee was concerned about the increase in overweight and the decrease in physical fitness levels among children. The hours that students spent inactively watching TV or playing with their computers and their propensity to choose foods with too much fat, salt, or sugar also were concerns. Some members worried about the number of students who engaged in physical activities like biking, in-line skating, and skateboarding without appropriate safety gear. After discussing their concerns, committee members decided to create a program that would involve both students and parents in improving their physical activity, nutrition, and safety habits.

The FIT 4 LIFE Program

The FIT 4 LIFE Program helps students, with the assistance of their families and teachers, record their daily healthy choices over a month-long period. Students are given a list of types and lengths of physical activity, healthy food choices, and good health habits, each of which earns them a certain number of points. In the case of physical activity, those points can be doubled if the student is active with another family member.

Examples of the points assigned to various activities appear in the following figure.

Physical Activities	20 min	40 min	60 min
Aerobics	6	8	10
Basketball	4	6	8
Cycling	4	6	10
Golf	1	3	5

Healthy Habits		
Brush teeth twice a day	1	
Wear your seat belt (each ride)	2	
Do a good deed without being asked	3	
Take a first aid or CPR class	10	

Nutrition		
Eat a healthy breakfast		2
Try a new nutritious food		1
Day without high-fat foods		2
Day without caffeine in drinks and no chocolate		2

Examples of FIT 4 LIFE fitness point assignments

Staff members are also invited to participate and talk to students about their own involvement. In this way, they can serve as role models for students.

Students submit their recording sheets to their teachers on a weekly basis at the elementary school level and at the end of the month in high school. At the end of the month, those students who have accumulated a set number of points receive FIT 4 LIFE award certificates. Each school sets the number of points that students must earn. This allows schools whose populations may differ, such as special education centers, to determine what is reasonable for their students.

Running and Promoting the Program

To start the program, the committee created masters of a brochure and a letter to be sent to families and staff to explain the program, an activity point list, a one-month recording sheet, and a certificate of recognition. These masters were handed out to a health and physical education teacher at each school, who could then duplicate them for their school's program. The teachers were given an orientation to the program and the materials at department chair meetings and at staff development workshops.

The committee also thought a 30-minute introductory video to the program might be helpful in explaining it to parents. To create the video, a subcommittee met with staff from the health and physical education office and the media center. The video included a moderator, two teachers, and two parents discussing the program. Their comments were interspersed with footage of families enjoying physical activities and of studio demonstrations of how to choose enjoyable activities and prepare nutritious snacks. The video was aired on the Fairfax County cable network channel, and it has been used in schools when staff first introduce the program to parents or students.

The health and physical education teachers in charge of the program chose various ways to introduce it. Some upper elementary teachers held assemblies; others presented it first to parents through the Parent Teacher Association. Middle and high school teachers gave out and explained the materials to students. Children in grades K through 4 were not included because they would not be able to do the necessary record keeping.

Program Results

Upper elementary school teachers who have used the program say that their students have been enthusiastic about working for the certificate. Students have encouraged their parents to work out with them so they can get the extra points. Parents have praised the school's effort to support healthy behaviors that the parents have been trying to work on at home, especially regarding nutrition and safety.

Upper elementary school teachers have found that running the program both in the fall and the spring allows more students to earn points for outdoor activities. If the program is conducted in the winter, the students who play on winter sports teams seem to have an edge.

Instructors teach nutrition education and personal health and safety lessons as part of the school health education curriculum. Because this fits so well with the FIT 4 LIFE program, classroom teachers have collaborated with physical education teachers in coordinating use of the program with the appropriate health lessons.

High school teachers report that students are interested in the program when it is made a part of health or physical education. It fits with the schools' activity-based health education unit, with units on aerobics and weight training, and with the physical education video series produced by the

American Alliance for Health, Physical Education, Recreation and Dance. FIT 4 LIFE can be used to help students achieve two of the physical education exit standards: "students to demonstrate competence in one self-selected lifetime sport or activity" and "students [to] develop a personal fitness action plan."

Both staff and parents have had many good things to say about the FIT 4 LIFE program. Future plans for the program are to add having students set a long-term wellness goal after the month's recording of activities, based on the information from that record.

Conclusion

FIT 4 LIFE has proven to be a simple but effective way of making both students and their parents more aware of what they can do to be healthier. The program is of little cost to the school and can be integrated into existing health and physical education classes, promoting collaboration between classroom and physical education teachers. During the month the program is in force, it promotes physical activity for students and their parents and reinforces students' knowledge of healthy behavior. This story illustrates how parents and school staff can collaborate to design a program that works well for both home and school.

Summary

The success stories shared in this book are quite diverse and clearly show that there's no one magic formula for increasing physical activity among young people. Still, some similarities among the stories are worth considering.

Perhaps the most important common factor to the stories we've shared in this book is that in every instance it was an individual who was willing to stick his or her neck out to make a difference, to try a new way, who served as the catalyst for change. Policy didn't get changed, new programs didn't get started, and additional space didn't get allocated until one concerned person started the ball rolling.

It should be further noted that these individuals started with their best effort, but continually modified what they were doing, throwing out what didn't work and keeping and expanding what did. They eventually brought in more people to help them, but in most cases this happened after the project was underway.

Examples of individuals who served as catalysts for change include Lee Allsbrook in Murfreesboro, TN (success story number 2), Caldwell Nixon, Lincolnton, NC (3), and Ernest Smith, San Diego, CA (6).

We hope you will be the person in your community who serves as a catalyst for change, and we hope the stories we've shared in this book will give you some ideas for getting started. The following are additional factors common to our success stories that we think are worth considering.

MEET THE INTERESTS OF YOUNG PEOPLE

Sometimes it's difficult for an adult to understand why young people don't enjoy the same physical activities he or she enjoys. It's not unusual for a physical education teacher or recreation leader, for example, to have been a competitive athlete in school and, partly as a result of this, offer traditional physical education and recreation programs that focus on competitive team and individual sports. However, not all young people like competitive sports, and these traditional curriculums have been a turn-off for many children and adolescents.

It is not surprising, then, that many of our success stories have involved innovative, varied activities that reflect the interests of young people. The health benefits of mountain biking are just as valuable as the health benefits from playing basketball. The key is getting young people physically active—and young people are much more likely to be active if they enjoy the activity.

When choosing activities for your program, several factors are very important to consider, including the ages of the young people you want to involve, their interests and abilities, their environment, and their cultural heritage. It works much better to fit the activities to the young people rather than trying to force the young people to fit the activities. Examples of programs meeting the ever-changing interests of students include the Cabell Midland High School Program (11), the Madison Junior High School Program (13), and the University Park Community Center (15).

Along with selecting appropriate activities that are motivating for students, you might also consider an incentive program to capture student interest. The idea is not to make the incentives the primary reason for being physically active but to use them to help get your new program up and running. The Fairfax County Schools FIT 4 LIFE Program (20) is an example of a program that successfully uses appropriate incentives.

DEVELOP QUALITY FIRST

From reading the success stories, it's clear that to gain support you first have to build a quality program and then go to others to share what you're doing and ask for support. This is not easy, but you need to show people what works rather than tell them it will work. Build the best program you can with the resources you have, and then show everyone in your community what you've done. You'll be much more likely to get their support for expanding and improving a program that is already successful. For example, if you have a poor physical education program with an outdated and inappropriate curriculum, it's unlikely you'll be able to convince the taxpayers in your community that you should add physical education teachers and expand the program. The first step is to improve the curriculum, involve others in the changes, and *then* look for expansion support.

The Clovis High School Program (1) is a great illustration of how a community will get behind a strong program. In the Arizona State University/ Mesa Elementary School Cooperative Physical Education Project (7), a top quality program was first developed, which then led to additional support. The work in developing Michigan's Exemplary Physical Education Curriculum Project (8) is another fine example of building a strong program first.

GET OTHERS INVOLVED

Earlier we said that it was action from a single individual that got our success stories started. However, these individuals quickly recruited others to support and promote their ideas. Programs have a much better chance of success once a wide base of support is gained. Asking others for ideas can help make them feel ownership of the program. If others feel they have a part in planning a project, they are far more likely to support that project.

Gaining support from the community were major factors in the success of the Forest High Campus SELF Center (5), the Clay Organized for Wellness Program (14), and the Stilwell Junior High Intramural Program (18).

KEEP PEOPLE INFORMED

People involved in the physical activity profession are rarely publicity hounds, but to gain widespread support for your program, you've got to get your positive news out to the community. Find ways of letting everyone in your community know about what you're doing and how your program is helping young people.

The Wellness Initiatives in Escambia County Schools (4), the Family Fitness Program (19), and the people involved in the Fairfax County Schools FIT 4 LIFE Program (20) all made sure they kept parents and other key people informed of what they were doing. Lee Allsbrook (2) involved the media in his fight to change policy.

ASSESS WHAT YOU'RE DOING

Assessment is important for several reasons. First, you need to assess what you are doing to know if you are reaching your objectives. The results of your assessments can help you improve your program. Second, assessment, when done well, enhances student learning. Third, providing assessment results to parents, taxpayers, administrators, and others will give them a better understanding of what you're accomplishing, making it easier to win their support.

The PATH Program (9) serves as an example of how you need to continually assess and improve a program once it has been started. Sue Schiemer and the Bloomsburg Area School District Program (10) have developed an outstanding assessment program. The Clay Organized for Wellness Program (14) shows the value of formative research in the development of a program.

INCLUDE EVERYONE

Physical activity can benefit *all* people regardless of their abilities or current physical condition. Develop a program that is inclusive and you'll find that previously inactive young people want to be involved—you'll also find increased support for your program.

The Minnesota State High School Adapted Athletic Program (17) is a good example of a program where students of all abilities benefit from physical activity.

MAXIMIZE RESOURCES

By maximizing resources, what we really mean is getting the "biggest bang for your buck." It's unlikely that you'll ever have an unlimited budget for your program—not even in the best case scenario. So it's vital that you make the best possible use of every penny and every resource you do have. This will not only increase the value of your current program but will also raise your chances of getting more resources for future programs by showing how well you are able to stretch a budget.

The Mitchell High School Adventure Education Program (12) and the University Park Community Center (15) programs are excellent examples of programs that maximize their resources.

NO EXCUSES

"Given what we know about the health benefits of physical activity, it should be mandatory to get a doctor's permission *not* to be active."

We've modified this quote, attributed to Per-Olof Astrand of the Karolinska Institute of Sweden, to sum up the theme of this book: *Given what we know about the benefits of physical activity for young people, and what we know about creating successful physical activity programs, it should be mandatory for community leaders to get a doctor's permission not to develop physical activity programs for young people in their communities.*

So, good luck—and remember that you're not alone. The people who contributed to this book are willing and able to help you with any questions you might encounter as you make a difference in your community.

Resources

A guide for the development of competency-based curricula for entry level health educators. 1983. New York: National Task Force on the Preparation and Practice of Health Educators.

Centers for Disease Control and Prevention. 1997. *Guidelines for school and community programs to promote lifelong physical activity among young people.* MMWR 46(No. RR-6):1-24.

Health instruction responsibilities and competencies for elementary (K–6) classroom teachers. 1992. *Journal of Health Education* 23 (6):352-54.

Healthy People 2000: National health promotion and disease prevention objectives. 1991. Washington, D.C.: U.S. Department of Health and Human Services, Public Health Service.

Joint Committee on National Health Education Standards. 1995. *National health education standards.* New York: American Cancer Society.

National Association for Sport and Physical Education. 1995. *Moving into the future: National physical education standards.* St. Louis: Mosby.

National Association for Sport and Physical Education. 1995. *National standards for athletic coaches: Quality coaches, quality sports.* Dubuque, IA: Kendall/Hunt Publishers Co.

National Association for Sport and Physical Education. 1995. *National standards for beginning physical education teachers.* Reston, VA: The Association.

National Association for Sport and Physical Education. 1994. *Sport and physical education advocacy kit.* Reston, VA: The Association.

Pale, R.R., M. Pratt, S.M. Blair, W.L. Haskell, C.A. Macera, C. Bouchard, D. Buchner, W. Ettinger, G.W. Heath, A.L. King, et al. 1995. Physical activity and public health. A recommendation from the Centers for Disease Control and Prevention and the American College of Sports Medicine. *JAMA* 273 (5):402-7.

U.S. Department of Health and Human Services. 1996. *Physical activity and health: A report of the surgeon general.* Atlanta, GA: U.S. Department of Health and Human Services, Centers for Disease Control and Prevention, National Center for Chronic Disease Prevention and Health Promotion.

On the state and local levels, you can obtain information about physical activity from the following groups:

- Affiliates of voluntary health organizations, such as the American Heart Association
- State and local health departments
- Your state's Governor's Council on Physical Fitness and Sports
- State associations of the American Alliance for Health, Physical Education, Recreation and Dance
- Organizations that serve young people, such as the YWCA

On the national level, information is available from the following agencies:

American Alliance for Health, Physical Education, Recreation and Dance
1900 Association Drive
Reston, VA 20191-1599
800-213-7193

American Cancer Society
1599 Clifton Road NE
Atlanta, GA 30329-4251
800-227-2345

American College of Sports Medicine
P.O. Box 1440
Indianapolis, IN 46206-1440
317-637-9200

American Heart Association
7272 Greenville Avenue
Dallas, TX 75231-4596
800-242-8721

American School Health Association
P.O. Box 708
Kent, OH 44240-0708
330-678-1601

National Association for Sport and Physical Education
1900 Association Drive
Reston, VA 20191-1599
800-213-7193, ext. 410

National Association of Governor's Councils on Physical Fitness and Sports
201 South Capitol Avenue, Suite 560
Indianapolis, IN 46225
317-237-5630

National Center for Chronic Disease Prevention and Health Promotion
Division of Adolescent and School Health Resource Room
Centers for Disease Control and Prevention
4770 Buford Highway NE, MS K-32
Atlanta, GA 30341-3724
888-CDC-4NRG

National Heart, Lung and Blood Institute Information Center
P.O. Box 30105
Bethesda, MD 20824-0105
301-251-1222

National Recreation and Park Association
2775 South Quincy Street, Suite 300
Arlington, VA 22206-2204
800-649-3042, 703-578-5558

President's Council on Physical Fitness and Sports
701 Pennsylvania Avenue NW
Suite 250
Washington, DC 20004
202-272-3421

More ideas for promoting lifelong health and fitness

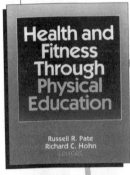
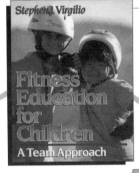
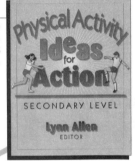
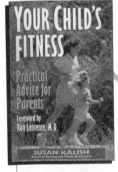
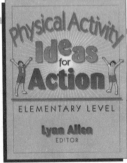